Mussar
YOGA

*Blending an Ancient
Jewish Spiritual Practice
with Yoga to Transform
Body and Soul*

EDITH R. BROTMAN, PHD, RYT-500

FOREWORD BY ALAN MORINIS,
founder and director, The Mussar Institute

For People of All Faiths, All Backgrounds
JEWISH LIGHTS Publishing

Mussar Yoga:
Blending an Ancient Jewish Spiritual Practice with Yoga to Transform Body and Soul

2014 Quality Paperback Original Edition
© 2014 by Edith R. Brotman
Foreword © 2014 by Alan Morinis

Library of Congress Cataloging-in-Publication Data
Brotman, Edith R.
  Mussar yoga : blending an ancient Jewish spiritual practice with yoga to transform body and soul / Edith R. Brotman, PhD.
      pages cm
  Includes bibliographical references and index.
    ISBN 978-1-58023-784-0 (quality pbk.) — ISBN 978-1-58023-801-4 (ebook) 1. Spiritual life—Judaism. 2. Yoga. 3. Self-realization—Religious aspects—Judaism. 4. Jewish ethics. I. Title.
  BM723.B735 2014
  296.7—dc23
                                2014009170

Manufactured in the United States of America
Cover Design: Jenny Buono
Cover Art: Shutterstock © Tshooter
Interior Design: Tim Holtz

For People of All Faiths, All Backgrounds
Published by Jewish Lights Publishing
An Imprint of Turner Publishing Company
4507 Charlotte Avenue, Suite 100
Nashville, TN 37209
Tel: (615) 255-2665
www.jewishlights.com

Contents

"Discovering the truth about ourselves is a lifetime's work, but it's worth the effort."

—**Fred Rogers**, *The World According to Mister Rogers*

Foreword

ALAN MORINIS

If not for yoga, I would not have found *Mussar.* Or, even if I had, I would not have recognized it as the precious spiritual path that it is. I had lived in India for three years exploring Hinduism and Buddhism, and it was in classes under the hawk-like gaze of yoga master B. K. S. Iyengar that I came to understand that each of us needs to take his or her own spiritual journey. In those yoga classes, we were all doing the same poses at the same time, but our teacher would focus each of our efforts on specific areas that he saw needed attention. I was strong and so he focused me on developing flexibility, whereas my wife was flexible and so she was made to work on building strength. No two people are alike, so spiritual practice needs to address the uniqueness of the individual.

It was many years later that twists in my life sent me on another spiritual search, this time within the Jewish world of my birth and upbringing. In my almost fifty years of encounter with the organized Jewish world, I hadn't seen much attention paid to individual distinctiveness. Everything Jewish seemed to focus on community, collective ritual, and common practices, with not much concern for the individual and his or her uniqueness. When I stumbled on writings about *Mussar*, it appeared to me to be the missing piece: a Jewish spiritual tradition that, like yoga, provides pathways of practice that are geared to the needs and the potential of the individual, not the collective.

It is apparent to the eye that we are distinct from one another in regard to our bodies, but we are just as dissimilar in our inner lives. Bringing together *Mussar* and yoga forms a single discipline that addresses both dimensions, the physical and the spiritual. Although *Mussar* teachers of previous centuries developed meditations, contemplations, visualizations, and chanting practices, there is no evidence of a discipline involving the body. Edith Brotman has filled in that missing piece with a practice that is true to both its parents.

The word for "wholeness" in Hebrew is *shlemut*. *Mussar* practice aims to help us become more *whole* in our lives. It is focused on helping us move from partialness or even brokenness toward wholeness. Yoga embodies a similar concept, called *purna* in Sanskrit. By marrying *Mussar* practice and yoga practice, this book opens a new pathway to developing greater wholeness.

The urge to develop our potential is seeded deep within the human soul. This book shows us that body and soul can be good partners for acting on and realizing that deep inner urge. The wholeness that comes of our efforts in turn affects both body and soul, and we experience the fruit of our efforts in the form of inner peace—*shalom*—a word that comes from the same linguistic root as *shlemut*. This book is a guide to becoming whole, body and soul, which is the only way I know to come to *shalom*.

Acknowledgments

T he seeds of this book were planted a very long time ago and thus many debts have accumulated along the way.

My editor, Emily Wichland, vice president of Editorial and Production at Jewish Lights, guided me through the writing process as the kind and knowledgeable professional that she is. Many thanks to Ally E. Machete at Ambitious Enterprises, who read many early drafts and offered very helpful comments.

Most of the credit for the book's photography belongs to Edward J. Winter Photography with models Melissa Daum, Eric Brown, and Michael Marion, who volunteered their time. Several photographs were also taken by Shawn Paterakis.

I am very grateful to Alan Morinis for his brilliant vision and dedication to taking up the mantle of Israel Salanter and the other masters of the *Mussar* movement by reviving and spreading *Mussar* to the broad audience it deserves. I am also grateful for his support and encouragement for the idea (if, perhaps, not all the content) of this book.

It's not an exaggeration to say that *Mussar Yoga* would never have come to fruition without the inspiration of Elka Abrahamson at the Wexner Foundation. I am also grateful for my Baltimore Wexner friends who agreed to be lab rats for my *Mussar* experiments, especially Jill Max, Melissa Cordish, Harel Turkel, Randi Buergenthal, Rachel Steinberg-Warschawski, Becky Brenner, and Jon Cardin. Thanks also to Yehuda Neuberger for his friendship. I am also indebted to Jennifer Meyerhoff and Michelle Rosenbloom, who first suggested that I create a written version of *Mussar* Yoga. The writing of this book was also supported through a Dorbrecht Grant for Judaic Yoga.

Many thanks to Daniel Matt, Steve Haddad, and Angela Jamison for their attempts to school me in the meaning of the traditional texts and concepts. In my sincere yet stubborn effort to build bridges between *Mussar* and yoga, I may have unintentionally corrupted the meaning of some of the teachings. I accept full responsibility for any accidental misrepresentations.

Much appreciation to Rabbi Andrew Busch for his helpful reading of early drafts and suggestions of sources of Jewish content. And sincere thanks to the other members of the Baltimore Hebrew Congregation community—Rabbi Elissa Sachs-Kohen, Andy Wayne, Brad Cohen, Cantor Robbie Solomon, Cantor Ann Sacks, and the Monday lunchtime yoga crew.

I am very grateful for my yoga family at Charm City Yoga (notably Kim Manfredi) for supporting my teaching of yoga and *Mussar* Yoga. Special thanks to Tami Schneider at Cleveland Yoga, whose teaching changed my life and made all the good things possible.

To my friends, students, and fellow teachers, especially Eva Allen, Lauren Flax, Kris Hare, and Jane and Michael Marion—you rock! To the military veterans with whom I have had the privilege to teach and share life's ups and downs, thank you. Steve LeVine deserves special thanks for his enthusiastic help doing whatever was needed—reading drafts, running errands, feeding my kids dinner, and reminding me to stay on task.

Love to my father, Robert Raphael (and through him to my great-grandfather, R. B. Raphael, a true Litvak scholar from whom I seem to have inherited the writer gene). Thanks also to my mother, Phyllis Rubinstein Raphael (*alev hashalom*), who handed down her own brand of intellectual seriousness.

Many thanks to my beloved husband, Daniel, for his love of the messy and unfinished project that is me and his unconditional support for this book.

To my beautiful children, Parker and Naomi. Thank you for being patient with the hours I am away attending board meetings, leading workshops and retreats, or sitting on a stool at Starbucks writing about Jewish spirituality. My love for you both is limitless and beyond words.

A Note to the Reader

To an outsider, yoga enthusiasts probably sound a bit like actors in an infomercial. Yoga, it seems, has liberated multitudes of people from physical or psychic pain, bad habits, addictions, emotional distress or disease, and even general malaise. Like some magic elixir, yoga appears to change people's lives and they can't stop talking about how great it is.

I am one of those true believers in the power of yoga. I've seen it transform people physically, making them stronger and more flexible. Their skin begins to glow and they look more relaxed. But the real magic of yoga is not about what happens on the mat. Yoga changes people because it uses the physical body as a gateway to making changes in the soul. Yoga works to uproot old negative patterns and replace them with more healthy practices.

The key to yoga's transformational abilities lies in its attention to the inner workings of the self. The self-awareness that happens *on* the mat paves the way for self-awareness *off* the mat. As soon as I realized how much energy I wasted worrying and judging others, for example, I became a better mother, wife, and friend. These days I worry less about the uncertain future and focus more on being present and compassionate. At the risk of sounding like a paid advertisement, I attribute my greatest accomplishments over the past fifteen years to yoga. Through yoga I have also become more patient and less reactive. The community and organizational leadership positions, the honors, the Dorbrecht Grant for Judaic Yoga, which helped fund the writing of this book, were all opened up to me through the practice. Even my journey into *Mussar*, a Jewish form of ethical self-inquiry, was forged through my experiences with yoga's emphasis on self-study. (All my deficits, of which there are still many, come from lapses in commitment to the practice.)

Through yoga I have come to *Mussar*, and with *Mussar* I found a bridge between my faith in yoga and my desire and commitment to live a Jewish life. *Mussar* also adds depth to my understanding of yoga and affirms my faith in the oneness of the Universe. I am very grateful to have discovered *Mussar*'s powerful use of mantras, journaling, and studying with a partner or in groups.

Mussar or yoga will not likely cure your psoriasis or keep termites from infesting your woodpile, but they can open up new universes of possibility. *Mussar* Yoga is one such "new universe of possibility." Just as someone figured out that peanut butter combined with chocolate forms a delicious treat, and now the combination seems ubiquitous, obvious, and altogether natural, the combination of *Mussar* and yoga feels similarly inspired. The blending of *Mussar*, which is rooted in Judaism, with yoga, which originated in South Asia, creates a transformational experience. If you're ready for change, *Mussar* Yoga will deliver it to you in a new and powerful way.

An important disclaimer: I am neither a rabbi nor a scholar of Judaics. My knowledge of *Mussar* is primarily self-taught. I am not fluent in either Hebrew or Sanskrit. When I read sacred texts, I read them in translation. No doubt, some in the *Mussar* and yogic communities will quibble or outright quarrel with my interpretations and the blending of concepts and practices. If you are seeking a pure or traditional approach to *Mussar* or yoga, this is not the book for you. The only thing pure in this book is my intent—to offer another vista on the journey of our souls.

The material for the book comes from the school of life viewed through the lens of more than a decade of practicing and teaching yoga, informal Jewish studies with rabbis and academic scholars, decades of teaching college sociology, and years of facilitating *Mussar* and *Mussar* Yoga workshops. Every day I learn more about yoga and *Mussar* through my children, husband, friends, and colleagues, who continually teach and challenge me.

Introduction

Everywhere you look these days people seem to be doing yoga—grandmothers, Marine Corps captains, toddlers, people in commercials for everything from cereal to life insurance, football players, even politicians. Generally, when people speak of yoga they are referring to Hatha yoga—the *asanas*, or poses, that are typically presented in yoga videos or classes. But this conception of yoga limits it to a form of exercise. Yoga is much more than exercise: It is a spiritual discipline in which the physical movements facilitate the spiritual journey. Yoga is shorthand for the Eight Limbs of Yoga that, as a whole, are meant to transform our relationship to other people, to other living things, and, ultimately, to the Divine Presence.

Mussar Yoga is a means of profound and lasting transformation that blends two spiritual practices from two different cultural traditions: Judaism and Vedic Brahamism. While yoga is widely popular, *Mussar* (pronounced muss-er or moos-AHR) is still relatively unknown, even among most Jews. *Mussar*, which can also be transliterated *Musar*, means "instruction" in Hebrew. This Jewish practice of self-study is similar in some ways to the yogic concept of *svadhyaya* (self-study). Both offer a strategy for following the timeless command to "know thyself." At its core, *svadhyaya* is "the drawing out of the best that is within [oneself]."[1] Likewise, *Mussar* asks: "Do you know what is necessary for your own perfection and what pertains to the relationship between you and your Maker ... from the standpoint of your heart and thoughts?"[2]

> *Mussar* means "instruction."

Mussar and Yoga: A Brief History

Yoga and *Mussar* grew out of larger religious traditions—yoga from Brahamism, the spiritual antecedent of Hinduism and Buddhism, and *Mussar* from Judaism. Yoga's language (Sanskrit) and its literature share roots with Hinduism, but its modern Western form strikes a universal chord. B. K. S. Iyengar and other leading yogis define yoga as a philosophy that promotes spirituality.[3]

The origins of *Mussar*, the name and the texts related to it, clearly belong to Judaism. The word *Mussar*, signifying inner instruction, appeared in Jewish writings, according to Alan Morinis, as far back as the eighth century CE. But for many centuries it was mainly the solitary pursuit of individuals while scholarship of the Hebrew Bible and oral laws (Talmud) took place in study groups and schools. Throughout the ages, *Mussar* had texts: *Duties of the Heart*, a seminal *Mussar* work written by Bachya ibn Paquda in Spain, appeared in the early eleventh century. In 1740, Rabbi Moshe Hayyim Luzzatto of Padua, a talented scholar of Kabbalah, moved to Amsterdam and published his influential *Mussar* text, *Path of the Just*.

The *Mussar* movement emerged in eighteenth-century Lithuania.

Also in the mid-eighteenth century, Benjamin Franklin, writing in geographically and culturally distant colonial Protestant America, proposed a system of self-improvement in which thirteen traits or virtues would be studied individually for one week (that is, one per week) for a total of thirteen weeks, in a cycle to be repeated four times a year.[4] Speculation exists that as Enlightenment spread slowly across Europe, Franklin's writing seeped into the intellectual awareness of Eastern European rabbis. About one hundred years after Luzzatto and Franklin's works appeared, Rabbi Israel Salanter, a brilliant and well-respected scholar based in Vilna, Lithuania, launched the *Mussar* movement. Salanter advocated not only studying ethical behavior, but also infusing the heart with virtue and cultivating habits of goodness.[5] Through Salanter and his disciples, *Mussar* became more formalized with texts, methodologies (including the cyclical study of thirteen traits), and, eventually, yeshivas (schools/academies). In a very short time, the *Mussar* movement spread, establishing various branches and schools of study in Germany and throughout Russia.

The strength of the movement was, however, no match for persecution by the Bolsheviks and then the Nazis. Most of the *Mussar* masters of the twentieth century and their students did not survive the Holocaust. Those who did helped incorporate *Mussar* into the curriculum of the Orthodox yeshivas in the United States and Israel. Thus, for much of the twentieth century, *Mussar* was relegated to a small corner of Orthodox Judaism, while the majority of Jews—Reform, Conservative, Reconstructionist, Renewal, and secular—had never heard of it.[6]

Today, *Mussar* is experiencing an exciting revival. *Mussar* study groups are popping up across the United States and even in Europe. Members of every branch of Judaism—Renewal, Reconstructionist, Reform, Conservative, and Modern Orthodox—are discovering new spiritual inspiration in *Mussar*. Secular Jews, drawn to Eastern practices, have begun turning to *Mussar* as a bridge between the two. *Mussar*, like yoga, taps into our collective desire to embark on an inner spiritual journey that leads us to a closer connection with the Divine. Indeed, the combination of the two into *Mussar* Yoga responds to the popular demand for powerful and universal spiritual tools.

Why Combine *Mussar* and Yoga?

It might seem that yoga, derived from Hinduism and Buddhism, and *Mussar*, steeped in Eastern European Jewish Orthodoxy, are a strange combination. Yet both respond to the universal desire to better ourselves and improve the world around us. Both approaches, informed by thousands of years of the wisdom of great sages, add their unique strengths to the challenges of life.

Yoga's code of ethics centers on ten virtues outlined by the sage Patanjali. One of the ten virtues is the discipline (*niyama*) called *svadhyaya*—self-study. B. K. S. Iyengar writes in his book *Light on Life* that *svadhyaya* involves "reading scripture and seeing their truths reflected in one's own life."[7] Similarly, *Mussar* directs students to look at themselves through the lens of Torah, Talmud, and the wisdom of rabbis and sages. *Mussar* materials include quotations from a range of Jewish sources, including the Hebrew Bible; the talmudic tractate on ethics, *Pirke Avot*; and the words of Rabbi Akiva, Maimonides, and sages of the Jewish mystical tradition, Kabbalah. Similarly, yoga, especially contemporary Western yoga, draws from a wide range of liturgy that adheres to universal themes of peaceful, truthful, and simple living while acknowledging and honoring a higher power. Yogis consult the Yoga Sutras and the Upanishads, but they also quote the writings of Sufi poets, Buddhist monks, Hopi elders, and mystics of all traditions.

Mussar and yoga also share similar understandings of the purpose of self-study in relation to the soul. Judaism sees the soul (*neshama* in Hebrew) as the unchanging expression of divinity within us, and yoga has the same understanding of the soul, called *jivatman* in Sanskrit. For students of *Mussar*, self-study allows the light of the divine soul to shine outward more brightly. For yogis, self-study illuminates the path inward toward the divine soul.

Likewise, both yoga and contemporary *Mussar* favor concrete experience over intellectualism. "Think less," says Baron Baptiste, founder of the popular Baptiste Power Yoga Institute.[8] When we are fully in the body, there is no space for the thinking mind. Alan Morinis, founder of the Mussar Institute, similarly advises the practitioner not to engage with *Mussar* "passively and intellectually."[9] He advises people to take the concepts and "chew on them, argue with them, compare them to other ideas, try them out on your friends."[10]

Complementary Practices

The nineteenth-century founders of the *Mussar* yeshivas promoted various strategies of study to make *Mussar* a real, felt endeavor. One famous school of *Mussar*, Slabodka, embraced a behavioral approach; another, Kelm, emphasized contemplative practices; a third, known as Novarodok *Mussar*, favored an experiential curriculum. (In fact, this last one, Novarodok *Mussar*, was known for its "storm the soul" methods. Novarodok academies would, for example, send students into grocery stores asking for nails or hardware stores asking for flour to cultivate their humility.)[11]

The hot power yoga that I typically teach and practice can at times feel like storming the soul with its humbling intensity. In some ways, yoga can be thought of as a fourth type of *Mussar* academy that advocates the power of the physical realm, as well as the contemplative realm, to take us closer to self and God. As California-based spiritual leader Rabbi Mike Comins writes in his book *Making Prayer Real*, "Engaging the body is the most dependable way of moving us from the left to the right side of the brain," thus moving from the analytical and logical to the emotional and intuitive.[12] World-renowned lecturer on Jewish thought and philosophy Rabbi Akiva Tatz similarly says, "The only path to the spiritual is through the medium of the physical."[13] Connecting *Mussar* with yoga forms a broad bridge between physical experiences and the emotional, energetic, and spiritual work that goes along with self-reflection and change.

> "The only path to the spiritual is through the medium of the physical."

The starting point of *Mussar* Yoga is the *Mussar* concept of balancing our soul traits (*middot* in Hebrew) as a means of manifesting our inner divinity. If the meaning of our lives is to serve and love others, as the early *Mussar* masters insisted, then soul traits are tools to serve and love most effectively. Soul traits are our ethical behaviors and attitudes—emanations of the Divine in whose image we are created—that shape our lives through our interactions with others.

Through *Mussar* Yoga a person can explore the physical (bodily) dimension of any *Mussar* trait, such as humility, generosity, enthusiasm, and gratitude, by practicing yoga. While a person studies the trait of order, for example, the yogic practice of breathwork, or *pranayama*, can be useful. Establishing order typically involves both an emptying of space and a filling of space. When we clean out our e-mail inbox, we are freeing up room for new e-mails to arrive. When we breathe, we must expel the unneeded carbon dioxide to make room for the oxygen that fuels our body. A yogic *vinyasa*, or flow, sequence, which links movement with breath, disciplines us to the sequencing (ordering) of breath—inhaling in upward, lengthening movements, and then exhaling in downward and contracting movements. Through yoga, the *Mussar* student experiences such immediate and positive physical benefits of breath order that he is likely to reason to himself that applying order to other parts of his life—for example, home or work—would be equally beneficial.

Moreover, when we create and maintain *Mussar*'s order, we invite the yogic principle of *saucha* (purity) into our consciousness. Cleanliness demands order. Maintaining order around space and time prompts us to invite more purity into our lives. When we create order in our physical lives, there can be more order and less chaos in our mental, emotional, and spiritual lives.

Is the *Mussar* Yoga Path for You?

Mussar Yoga is a practice for anyone who wants to create new and better habits of being and living through (1) a method of self-discovery and improvement and (2) a system that works with the whole self—body, mind, and spirit. It is aimed at people who identify themselves as "spiritual seekers" and those who are but don't know it yet. Both experienced yoga practitioners and novices will feel comfortable and challenged by *Mussar* Yoga. If you are new to yoga, this book offers step-by-step instructions, helpful photographs, and resources for furthering your yoga practice. If you are already a practictioner of yoga, you will find that adding *Mussar* to your yoga will expand and transform your practice both on and off the mat.

Fundamentally, what is needed is an open mind, a bit of courage, and a willingness to shake up the status quo within you. The curriculum of *Mussar* Yoga works because it engages people on multiple levels. Are you someone who learns best by intellectually chewing over material? Or are you someone who needs a more physical, even tactile, approach? Are you self-motivated or do you need the company of others to keep you accountable, or a little bit of both? Whatever your answers are, *Mussar* Yoga meets you in your strengths and challenges you in your weaknesses. What kind of transformation does *Mussar* Yoga facilitate? It offers a way of living that is more in line with your purest motives and intentions in your relationships with others and with yourself. It cultivates the skills you need to gain greater awareness of your current habits of behavior and then, with kindness, assess whether those patterns are working for you or not. These skills and tools of self-inquiry and change come from the purposeful activities you engage in with yoga and *Mussar*, such as meditation, physical movements, directed breathing, repetition of phrases, and journaling.

The path of *Mussar* Yoga, like any good adventure, offers moments of both joy and challenge. If you are already a practitioner of yoga, especially if you have been treating yoga simply as a form of exercise, you might find that adding *Mussar* to your practice feels awkward at first. If you are new to yoga, getting into some of the poses may prove to be very challenging until your body gets stronger and more flexible. As with all new endeavors, stick with it for a period of time. "Life begins at the end of your comfort zone" is a common yoga refrain. The eighteenth-century mystic and visionary Rabbi Nachman of Breslov wrote, "All the world is a narrow bridge—the important thing is not to be afraid." Reb Nachman wants us to recognize that, from birth to death, life is full of change, and that change forces us to confront our fear of the unknown. The goal of *Mussar* Yoga is to free us from established patterns of being in order to live more fulfilling and meaningful lives.

Practicing *Mussar* Yoga requires bravery, a willingness to let go of our conditioned habits of living, and patience. It's a lifetime of practice. You will make progress on your journey and sometimes you will feel like you have lost your way or fallen off the path. But

Judaism and yoga (think of Moses and Buddha) teach us that each of those moments—the forward progress and the wandering—are part of the spiritual journey. Even better, once you take the first step on the path, the path becomes wherever you place your feet. So whether you are a seasoned yogi, a *Mussar* master, neither, or both, the path leads this way ...

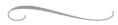

How to Practice
Mussar Yoga

I can't pretend to be a lion able to conquer the enemy,
To master myself would be enough.
I am only the dust on my Lover's path
and from dust I will rise and turn into a flower.

Rumi

Most of us have the feeling that we could be more—more loving, kind, organized, spiritual, disciplined, generous ... the
list goes on and on. We yearn to, as thirteenth-century Persian poet
Rumi writes, rise from the dust of our daily stumbling and bloom
into something fully beautiful.

We have the desire, but something is holding us back. The status quo may not be pleasant, but it has its advantages; the familiar
is, if nothing else, predictable and comfortable, the path of least
resistance. Maybe it is willpower, the strength to overcome the
power of habit. Maybe we do not specifically understand what we
need more of in our lives. Maybe we have a clear vision of what is
needed, but do not know how to get it.

How can we transform our life in a meaningful way? How do
we make real and lasting changes in our life? These are the questions that inspire the practice of *Mussar* Yoga.

B. K. S. Iyengar wrote, "If we can understand how our mind and
heart works [sic], we have a chance to answer the question, 'Why
do I keep making the same old mistakes?'"[1] In order to change,
then, we first need information, but we also need techniques.

Specifically, we need greater awareness of our current way of being and a strategy for change. One without the other will not bring us the change we seek.

The cross-cultural roots of *Mussar* Yoga provide an age-tested, successful formula for transformation through awareness and accountability. The exploration begins with an acute awareness or accounting of how the various soul traits play out in our lives. The more awareness we have going into the process, the more likely we will already know where our work lies. There are, however, likely to be surprises along the way. We may think, for example, that we have mastered the trait of silence by practicing silent meditation for an hour every day and taking extreme care not to dominate group discussions. But as we look for greater awareness, we may find that we are, in fact, prone to being too silent—failing to speak up to come to another's defense or using silence to emotionally distance ourselves from others. The first powerful tool of *Mussar* Yoga practice comes through the cultivation of truthful awareness.

Awareness: How Do You Measure Up?

What makes someone a good person? What qualities bear witness to the Divine within? And how well do we embody and express them in our daily lives? Benjamin Franklin and the *Mussar* masters of Eastern Europe believed that right living could be distilled down to thirteen soul traits or virtues. Which traits? Between the agnostic-secularist Franklin and the Orthodox rabbis there is some minor quibbling about labels and language, some deeper disagreement about how those traits show up in daily living, and certainly deep schisms around the relationship between religion and moral development. Nonetheless, they agreed that transformation begins with self-study—deep probing within—to determine how you currently live your life, focusing on the presence and strength of thirteen traits that promote humility, self-restraint, peaceful relations with others, and moderation in all endeavors and with the material world.

The thirteen specific traits (*middot*) of *Mussar* Yoga are truth, courage, humility, order, nonjudgment, zeal, simplicity, equanimity, generosity, silence, gratitude, loving-kindness, and trust. The following thirteen chapters are devoted to each of the traits in turn. These thirteen traits stand alone and follow no particular order. You can read the chapters in any order that appeals to you. There is overlap, of course: Generosity has much in common with loving-kindness, and humility ventures into the area of nonjudgment. One could convincingly argue for more than these thirteen, but working on these thirteen traits for a year or two is a good place to start.

A yoga practice increases self-awareness by reflecting, like a mirror, your inner emotional habits. The physical practice unmasks the nonphysical, peeling back the layers of being to reveal your patterns of reaction and expression. Power Yoga teacher Baron Baptiste observes that whatever emotions and reactions show up for you on the mat also show up in every other part of your life—in relationships, jobs, leisure time, and even moments of solitude. Who you are in Wheel Pose is who you are in a traffic jam, and that's the same person you are lying on a beach in paradise.[2]

As yoga reflects like a mirror, *Mussar* enlarges and clarifies like a microscope. You slide slices of your life under the powerful lens of *Mussar* and then adjust the view to see what is not typically seen with the naked eye. The thirteen traits tell you exactly where to focus your gaze. Just as pathologists know which cells to examine and which to ignore, *Mussar* instructs on how to look at your inner life. You set the lens to magnify how generosity plays out in the carpool line and with the homeless man on the street. Or how courage eludes you in your career or your relationships. The more you train yourself to observe your internal life, the more sensitive you become as your own witness. What previously slipped by unnoticed—the silly lie meant to cover your own embarrassment, the way you pass judgment on the mother with crying children in the neighborhood market, the small tug of resistance to changing your daily routine or meeting someone new—now pokes at your consciousness like a tack through the sole of your shoe.

> Mussar enlarges and clarifies like a microscope.

Mussar Yoga then offers the mirror, the microscope, and the checklist. The mirror to reflect back to you what is going on inside, the microscope for you to zero in on the particulars of your inner life, and the checklist to keep your quest focused. After you shift your vision and look deep within, you can begin to see where the work of reconciliation—between who you are and who you are meant to be—must begin.

Accountability: From Awareness to Action

Once we can see what our spiritual work entails, we can begin to hold ourselves accountable for getting it done. A good system of accountability is essential because our natural tendency is to slide back to the comfortable status quo. We may observe that our ego gets the best of us sometimes, vow to change, and for a few days or weeks seem to make progress. But after some time has passed our resolve begins to crumble. Unless we have a structurally sound system for supporting our best intentions, we'll soon find ourselves back where we began.

One wonderful feature of *Mussar* Yoga is that it offers many approaches and tools of accountability. The overall formula of *Mussar* Yoga study is to focus almost exclusively on one trait per week. Beyond that simple prescription there are many techniques from which to choose. First, *Mussar* Yoga can be practiced either alone or in groups. Studying with others can enhance both awareness and accountability. Listening to others grapple with a trait may open new doors of your own self-perception. Someone's observation about himself could spark a new insight for you. A productive group may also be able to make objective and compassionate observations about your relationship with a trait.

> **One trait per week for thirteen weeks, repeated four times a year.**

When you work with others, you have the accountability of designated meeting times and some degree of peer pressure to stay on top of your game. Knowing that you need to show up in person or in the virtual world on a particular day is motivating. When I lead *Mussar* Yoga workshops, I encourage participants to stay in contact with each other as much as possible between each session.

If you're practicing alone, you, the student, have more freedom to customize the order of the traits and to work on what is immediately relevant to your life. You might notice, for example, that you have had a string of forgotten appointments and want to work on getting better organized. You can put the trait of order in the queue for the coming week. A solitary practice is perfect for people who travel frequently for work or during the summer vacation months, when convening with others on a regular basis is just not practical or possible.

Second, *Mussar* Yoga includes a variety of techniques in its toolbox. The techniques work on different levels of experience—intellectual, physical, mental/emotional, and experiential. The intellectual piece comes from reading and studying the background of the trait and its various potential manifestations in your life. Each chapter begins with some background information. The trait of zeal, for example, begins with an exploration of two Hebrew words, *zerizut* and *zehirot*, which mean "enthusiasm" or "alacrity" and "diligence," respectively. Intellectually, then, we can begin to unpack the layers of meaning of this trait as enthusiastic commitment.

Engage intellectually.

The yoga component brings with it the opportunity to explore the physical embodiment of a trait. We can cultivate compassion or loving-kindness by doing heart openers (backbends), or we can feel the courage of vulnerability in Triangle Pose with our throat and vital organs open and exposed. Each chapter offers several yoga poses. Some chapters also incorporate breathing techniques (*pranayama*) and meditation practices that can help create a physical expression or experience of a trait.

Another successful technique of *Mussar* Yoga involves experiential work—taking your trait work into the world. A student practicing generosity, for example, commits to picking up the tab when having dinner with a friend or volunteering in a soup kitchen. Or perhaps she agrees to say "no" to more volunteer work because she has been too generous in the past and needs to spend more time with her family. Every chapter offers suggestions on how to deliberately pursue real-world experiences that can help inform and challenge you in relation to that particular trait. When working with silence, for example, you will be asked to consider the circumstances under which you are most prone to engage in gossip.

Each of the following thirteen chapters also provides one or more mantras—short groups of words meant to be repeated—that remind us to redirect our attention to the trait work. Pick one of the mantras provided or select another phrase that means something to you. The words can be anything that remind you of your trait work, such as song lyrics, Bible verses, popular sayings, or folk ditties. For example, if you're trying to be more generous, you could choose the mantra "Give till it hurts." Or if you need to cut back, you could say, "Charity begins at home." Stick with one mantra for the week, writing it on a notecard or post-it note to put in one or more visible or meaningful locations. Some folks put a notecard by the bathroom sink so they can silently repeat the mantra while they brush their teeth. Others might post it by their computer or phone to remind them of the mantra at pivotal moments—such as being more compassionate to others while communicating on the Internet or by phone.

Engage physically.

Finally, every chapter concludes with questions for journaling, group discussion, meditation, or reflection. Each of these practices is a helpful way to stay in the practice. Journaling, meditation, and reflection can be incorporated into your daily routine. Alan Morinis, author of *Climbing Jacob's Ladder*, suggests that jotting down instances in your day where your trait work emerges is a useful tool in the beginning of your *Mussar* work.[3] Journaling works best if you get in the habit of writing at a particular time of day, every day, such as before bed. If you are studying *Mussar* Yoga with a group, it is helpful to check in with each other at designated times to support each other's efforts. Many of my groups send out a midweek reminder e-mail to stay mindful of the week's work.

Getting Started

As noted before, *Mussar* Yoga works on a thirteen-week cycle. Each trait is practiced for one week before you move on to another trait. Some weeks you may be tempted to extend the trait work for another week—perhaps you were making enormous progress, or just the opposite, you were so busy that you hardly paid any attention to the trait. As enticing as it may be to go another week, I have found that keeping to the one-week cycle works best. We want to work each trait with our greatest energy. When we extend beyond a week, our interest and resolve begin to wane, the freshness of the trait dwindles, and we will likely find ourselves falling back on old habits. It's akin to eating the same food at every meal. As much as we think that spinach is healthy, we need a varied diet and we risk growing tired of its taste after too many spinach smoothies, salads, and quiches.

Another important related concept of *Mussar* Yoga is moderation. Each trait manifests on a continuum between extremes. Equanimity, for example, stands between hyperreactivity and indifference. We should strive to moderate our reactions but not become indifferent to the world's problems. For the other traits as well, we need to be wary of imbalances. Truth, zeal, generosity, and order can be dangerous when taken to extremes. Yoga poses that emphasize balance can help us remember the importance of finding our center. Many arm balances require us to counterweight our heavy head with an opposite movement of the hips (if head draws back, hips pull forward). Other balancing poses simply depend on complete alignment of the body: that is, stacking the weight of all our parts into one straight center line.

Engage experientially.

Week to week, commit to engaging with the traits on an experiential level. Don't try to be too clever or intellectual about the material, parsing meanings too deeply or looking for the exception to every rule. Get out of your head and let your heart and soul take the reins. There is wisdom within you. Let your inner knowing percolate to the surface of your understanding of each trait. Keep the work personal. Put and keep yourself in the practice. There's an elegance and simplicity to the actions of your day-to-day life. Are you following through on your commitments or not? Is your house in order or not? If not, which rooms or spaces need attention? Get specific.

Preparation is also key. Besides a copy of this book, you might find it helpful to gather or arrange for a few other items for your *Mussar* Yoga journey:

- a yoga mat (perhaps a yoga block or strap as well)
- a journal (unlined art books work nicely) and a pen
- a designated space to meditate and practice yoga
- a list of which trait or traits to begin with
- a familiarity with some basic yoga knowledge

The Fundamentals of Yoga

Yoga poses can be practiced in two approaches: flow (also called *vinyasa*) and nonflow (such as Iyengar and Anusara styles of yoga). In flow yoga, the practitioner moves or flows from one pose into another in sequential fashion, while in nonflow each pose is entered and then exited the same way. For example, in flow yoga, a yogi typically moves from Forward Fold to Plank to Low Push-up to Upward Facing Dog to Downward Facing Dog to Warrior I as part of the Sun Salutation B sequence. In nonflow, a yogi would move from Mountain Pose to Warrior I and then return back to Mountain, before moving to the next standing pose. Because nonflow is generally more accessible for beginners, the instructions in this book tend to follow a nonflow style.

Use caution: Please keep in mind that although there are many health benefits that come from practicing yoga, it is always possible to injure yourself if you are not careful or if you do not follow the instructions correctly. The instructions contained in this book are mainly designed for a beginner with average physical ability.

Some poses, however, are targeted to more experienced yoga students with above-average physical ability. It is important to carefully determine whether some poses are not in your present range of ability. If you have physical limitations, are pregnant, or have a preexisting injury or medical condition, use extra caution and consult with a physician before attempting the postures on your own. Although young children may engage with *Mussar* and yoga, this book is most appropriate for teenagers and adults who are in relatively good physical and emotional health.

You should observe a few specific cautions as well. If you have high blood pressure, a detached retina, or an ear infection, you should avoid inverted poses (where the head is lower than the heart). Some teachers do not recommend inverted poses for women who are menstruating. For pregnant women, caution is advisable, although for most women all poses are safe during the first trimester. After that, consult with your physician. If you suffer from a herniated or slipped disk, do not attempt backbending poses.

There are five foundational poses from which you can enter into almost every other yoga pose. It will be helpful to familiarize yourself with the essential alignment points in these five poses before proceeding with the book.

Easy Pose
Suhkasana

In preschools around the country, Easy Pose is called "crisscross applesauce." But what seems easy for children (sitting on the floor) can be challenging for adults accustomed to sitting in chairs all day.

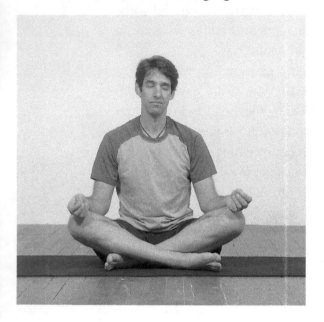

1 If you cannot remember the last time you sat comfortably on the floor, you might want to enlist the help of a blanket for a few weeks. Place a blanket (folded as necessary) under your hips so that your hips are slightly elevated.

2 Bend your knees and cross your legs. From time to time, switch which of your two legs is in front of the other.

3 Keep your spine long but not rigid. Open your chest and lift your chin parallel with the mat. Pull your ears back until they align over your shoulders.

4 Relax your hands on your thighs or kneecaps—palms faceup or facedown. Most seated poses can be entered from Easy Pose.

Mountain Pose
Tadasana

In yoga, Mountain Pose is considered *the* foundational pose—the points of alignment appear in essentially every other pose. In *vinyasa* yoga, Mountain Pose begins the Sun Salute sequences, which form the basis of flow. As you'll see, in nonflow traditions, Mountain is the starting and finishing stance for most standing poses.

Alignment for Mountain Pose begins at the base and builds its way up. What seems like simple standing is not. Because Mountain Pose is fundamental to all other poses, it comes with many alignment instructions.

1 Begin with the soles of your feet firmly rooted into the floor (without gripping your toes). Your feet are straight, hip-width apart (lining up with the outer edge of your hips), and your toes are pointed straight ahead. Gently rock back onto your heels and forth onto your toes a few times and then settle into the middle distribution point of your weight across your feet.

2 Hug your calf muscles into the surrounding bones and feel an energetic lift of your kneecaps.

3 Align your hip bones over your ankles and drop your tailbone into a neutral position (neither tucked too far forward—pushing your hip bones forward—nor lifted up too high, causing a sway in your lower back).

4 Pull your belly just below the belly button in and upward (called *uddiyana bandha*, or belly lock). For more precision, also contract and lift your pelvic-floor muscles (into what is called *mula bandh*, pelvic floor lock, or Kegel).

5 Draw your bottom rib cage slightly down toward the top of your hips.

6 Your spine is straight but not rigid and your shoulders stack on top of your hips as you drop them down away from your ears.

7 Pull your shoulder blades downward and slightly together.

8 Lift your chin off your chest so that your natural gaze is straight ahead. Draw your ears slightly back to align over your shoulders.

9 Lift your neck long. Soften the muscles around your lips and eyes.

Forward Fold
Uttanasana

Forward Fold is a motion as well as a pose. The motion of folding begins with the torso upright (as in Mountain Pose). The fold is often described as a "hinging of the hips." Like a lid on a hinge, the torso lowers (and rises) without any other movement in the body. In particular, the weight in the feet stays centered (rather than shifting back into the heels) and the hips stay lifted (rather than dropping down).

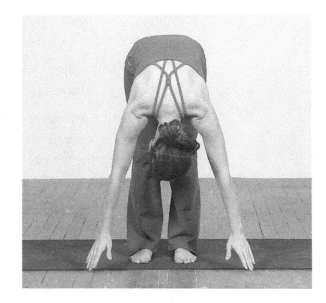

1 Begin in Mountain Pose. The first few times you try this pose, place your hands on your hips with your four fingers in the grooves just below your hip bones and your thumbs on the back of your hip bones. (Later you can come into this pose from a raised-arm position).

2 Tilt your torso forward while keeping your spine just as long as it was while standing upright. Reach the crown of your head forward. Take care not to let your shoulders fall forward or to let your back round.

3 You can soften your knees, allowing them to bend, but keep lifting your tailbone high.

4 Release your hands onto a block or the floor.

5 Drop the crown of your head toward the floor, releasing any tension in your neck.

Downward Facing Dog
Adho Mukha Svanasana

In flow yoga, Downward Facing Dog, which looks like an inverted "V," is the home pose. When you first learn it, you usually find it uncomfortable until you gain more strength and learn to minimize the pressure on your wrists. With enough practice, repetition, and attention to the alignment of your hands, Downward Facing Dog will become a resting pose.

1 Begin on your hands and knees with your hands slightly forward of your shoulders and your knees slightly behind your hips.

2 On an inhalation lift your knees off the mat and your hips high. On your next exhalation, drop your heels toward the mat.

3 Keep your hands and wrists forward of your elbows and your elbows forward of your shoulders. Press down into your bottom knuckles and finger pads, particularly your pointer finger and thumb. Feel an energetic lift in the heel of your hand.

4 Keep your hips high and forward of your knees and ankles.

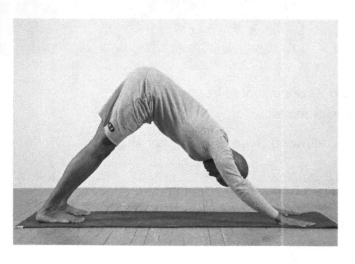

5 Gently press your chest toward your thighs, while keeping a lift in your armpits (i.e., not collapsing into the shoulder joints).

6 Align your ears between your arms, with the crown of your head pointed toward the floor. Keep all four sides of your neck long.

Warrior II
Virabhadrasana II

Warrior II is technically not a starter pose, as it typically is entered from either Mountain Pose or Downward Facing Dog. Warrior II, however, is a foundational pose for many of the poses in the Warrior series that are included in this book, such as Reverse Warrior (chapter 8), Bound Extended Side Angle (chapter 8), Half Moon (chapter 3), and Triangle (chapter 2).

1 To enter Warrior II from Mountain Pose, step your left foot to the back of the mat, leaving about three to four feet between your feet.

2 Leaving your left heel at the six o'clock position, turn your left toes to nine o'clock.

3 Pivot your torso to the left so that your hips and shoulders are square (on the same plane) to the left.

4 Raise and extend your arms to shoulder height and turn your head to gaze over your right fingertips. Draw your shoulder blades together and down your back.

5 Warrior II is a hip opener. Be sure to keep your hips level (drop your left hip, if necessary) and rotate your right thigh muscles clockwise behind you.

6 To protect your knees, make sure your right knee is directly above your ankle and that it points over your middle toes (not your big toe or to the left of your big toe).

With these five poses, considerations, and equipment items, you are ready to begin a journey of your soul. As with all journeys, once you start you never step off the path. You may encounter diversions, endless delays (as I write this, my *Mussar* partner texted to reschedule our meeting this afternoon), setbacks, frustrations, doubts, and fears. But in the end these are just an experiential part of the practice; they're another test to help you assess what work remains to be done.

The premise of *Mussar* Yoga is not that people can be perfect. Perfection is not the goal of our work. Our work is to improve and to reflect more clearly and brightly the divine light of our souls. Go forth and shine!

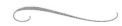

1

Truth

Stay far away from falsehood.

Exodus 23:7

If the mind thinks thoughts of truth, if the tongue speaks
words of truth and if the whole life is based on truth,
then one becomes fit for union with the Infinite.

B. K. S. Iyengar

Truth is the beginning of every good thing, both
in heaven and on earth; and he who would be
blessed and happy should be from the first a
partaker of truth, for then he can be trusted.

Plato

Hebrew: *emet*

Sanskrit: *satya*

Truth is a quality of being with others and with ourself and is
a foundational trait of *Mussar* Yoga. To effect real change, we
must first conduct an inventory of our current habits and patterns

of being. *Mussar* Yoga study begins with an honest accounting of who we are, what we do, and how we relate to others.

Both yoga and *Mussar* command us to be truthful. In Hebrew, the word for "truth" is *emet*, and it is reflected in the commandment not to bear false witness. In Patanjali's Eight Limbs of Yoga, truth, called *satya*, is one of the ten disciplines and restraints.

In our lives we can have three types of relationships with truth.

1. We can run away from it (but ultimately it has a way of catching up with us).
2. We can passively accept it when it arrive in our laps.
3. We can actively seek it out.

At their core, *Mussar* and yoga demand the last one—the relentless pursuit of truth and the willingness to honor truth in thoughts, words, and deeds, no matter how painful or difficult. A person cannot deal in falsehoods with others and have any sense of inner truth. The reverse holds equally true.

If we do not know already, *Mussar* Yoga study will make it clear that pursuing truth is a challenge. In her book *The Yamas and Niyamas*, author and yogi Deborah Adele writes that "the jewel of *Satya*, or truthfulness, isn't safe, but it is good."[1] We must approach truth with a fair amount of caution and respect for its power. There is nothing simple about it. We must engage truth with heightened awareness about our motives, feelings, and habits of being.

Why We Lie

Why don't we deal in truth? Perhaps we don't know what the truth is, or we don't want to know. Or perhaps we know, but the truth appears to conflict with another virtue, such as loving-kindness, or it is coupled with a vice, such as greed. In essence, fear or the pursuit of profit drives us from living in truth.

Our fear of the truth arises because truth can be painful, disruptive, dangerous, and destructive. We can think of our fear of truth as "pain avoidance." We presume that the pain of the truth outweighs the pain of lying and getting caught (or we presume we won't get caught). We may have done something wrong and are afraid of the penalty. It's easier for a child to blame the dog for the broken lamp than to deal with the punishment. As we get older, we may be afraid to admit to ourself that we are spending too much and saving too little because we're afraid to make the hard choices about where money is spent.

We might be inclined to stop with fear, but there is another primary motive to lying: profit. We might not fear the truth as much as we find profit in lying. Some people make calculated and rational decisions to lie and cheat because lying and cheating can yield substantial gain in financial, emotional, or other currency. Cheating on taxes is almost the norm. Even a wealthy parent may instruct a child to lie about her age in order to get a reduced rate at the zoo or amusement park.

If we want to polish our souls, though, we need to face our fears and place more value on truth than on short-term profit. Lies tend to beget lies. How, for example, does a parent explain to a child that it's okay to lie about her age for profit at the movie theater but not for profit on other occasions? Some Torah commentators have observed that the patriarch Jacob, who deceived his blind father, Isaac, in order to steal the birthright from his brother Esau, was then himself the victim of several painful deceptions.[2] When we engage in lying, we may inadvertently give other people permission to lie to us.

Again, truth may feel like a difficult trait. Truth may feel slippery and subjective. The Talmud devotes many tractates to teasing out when it is permissible to lie, including the well-known discussion about what to say to an unattractive bride on her wedding day and how it is permitted to lie when your life is in imminent danger. Others argue that the truth is very simple, a path to follow where at each fork we inquire of ourself, "True or not true?" and then follow the path of truth. The following pages in this chapter offer highlights from the wisdom of yoga and *Mussar* to help guide our practice of truth.

To Thy Own Self Be True

Living a more truthful life begins with being more truthful with ourself about ourself. *Mussar* Yoga encourages us to be more present, emotionally aware, and dedicated to discovering our path in this life.

An important skill in the *Mussar* Yoga approach to truth is learning to be true to your reality in the present moment. What is happening now? You are reading a book. While you have been reading, did your mind wander to a past event or a thought about future plans? Did you lose yourself in the stories about past and future? Perhaps you got caught up in anger over something that happened years ago or you fell into an enticing fantasy. Pursuing your own truth means that you need to learn to quiet the mind in order to distinguish reality from the thoughts in your head. As many yoga and meditation teachers have taught, life is only happening in the present moment. Everything else is not real or true. You may find profit in distracting yourself from the mundane elements of life, but too much distraction and denial has ill effects. The more you indulge in stories, the more you lose sight of what is real and present. The pursuit of truth requires vigilance.

Along with attending to the present moment, self-truth requires us to stay aware of our emotions. Baruch Spinoza, the seventeenth-century Jewish-Dutch philosopher, wrote, "Emotion, which is suffering, ceases to be suffering as soon as we form a clear and precise picture of it."[3] In the *Mussar* Yoga workshops I run, we begin each session with the following phrase: "Hi, I'm [name]. I pledge my confidentiality to the group and right now I am feeling [one of twelve core emotions]." Most of the participants need a few

Truth as awareness.

minutes to identify their current emotional state. It's interesting that many of us, except in times of extremes, have trouble labeling our emotions at any given moment. What we are not aware of may sabotage us. If we are not aware of our hurt or anger—and fail to address it directly—we may end up actively lashing out or becoming passively resentful. We can practice being more truthful to ourself by taking one moment every day to become aware of our specific feelings.

Finally, we move closer toward our truth by being authentic. Most of us have a desire to please others in one way or another. Sometimes this desire means that we are not staying true to our authentic selves. We are trying to be who we think other people—our parents, partner, friends, employer, and community—want us to be. Both yoga and *Mussar* teach that our role in this world is to fulfill our divinely ordained potential. Rabbi Menushalum Zusya said, "In the coming world they will not ask me, Why were you not Moses? They will ask me, Why were you not Zusya?"[4]

Be True to Others: Six Guidelines

In your dealings with others, truth can be a tricky virtue. You can either approach it with a raft of qualifications or you can take an absolutist approach that a person should tell the truth no matter what. *Mussar* Yoga strikes a balance by offering some general guidelines for being truthful.

1. Be True but Kind

As Deborah Adele notes, being truthful with others is not a form of self-indulgence. Instead, yoga teachers often refer to a three-layer sieve of self-expression. Each time we speak, we should filter our words through these questions: Is it true? Is it kind? Is it necessary? Only when our speech passes all three tests should we open our mouths.

Each of us is confronted by the actions of another that bother us on one level or another. I once had a student in my yoga class who broke many of the discipline's rules about cleanliness (*saucha*). His behavior sometimes turned my stomach and I'm sure others felt the same way. Likewise, a student in my *Mussar* group was disturbed by the behavior of his wife's friends who routinely mistreated the waitstaff at restaurants. When we are paying attention to being truthful, what do we do with the rude friends or the unclean student? The path of *Mussar* Yoga is that whatever we decide to say, it must be truthful, it must be kind, and we must feel that it is absolutely necessary. As long as we stay alert to and aware of those three rules, we can address these types of circumstances. In the case of the student, when I approached the situation from a place of kindness, I realized that he may not know how to clean his mat or that there is a box of tissues in the room for that purpose. I made a general announcement to the class on the basics of mat cleaning and other hygienic tips to keep everyone healthy.

2. Beware the So-Called White Lie

A white lie is one in which, in the name of being kind, we lie. A classic talmudic discussion addresses the moral conundrum of truth and the unattractive bride. On her wedding day, the bride—your best friend or your cousin's daughter—looks terrible. Social convention dictates that you tell the bride that she is beautiful. If you are living in a place of truth, you should be careful to be kind while remaining truthful. Remember from the story of the biblical Jacob that lies beget lies. White lies are quick fixes, instead of the doing the hard work of introspection and awareness. For example, instead of resorting to a white lie in speaking to the bride, if you take some time to explore your true feelings you can learn to see different types of beauty. Perhaps the bride and her dress are unattractive, but you can see her face glow with happiness. Or maybe her face is not glowing, but you can see how the groom looks at her with love.

3. Avoid Exaggeration, Hyperbole, and Extreme Superlatives

In a world where everyone is vying for attention, it is tempting to use extreme language to get others to notice what you are saying or doing. You compromise your own ability to communicate effectively and command authority if you label everything with words like *awesome* and *amazing.*

4. Be Honest in Your Business Dealings

The Talmud states that the first question a person is asked in the afterlife is this: "Were you honest in your business dealings?" (BT *Shabbat* 31a). Business is a realm fraught with temptations to lie and cheat. The lines between lying and creative business practices can easily get blurred.

5. Realize That Sometimes Truth Must Be Its Own Reward

A Canadian friend of mine regularly visits Israel and the territories, where she teaches yoga to Israelis and Palestinians in an effort to promote peace. On each return trip, she admits to security officials that she traveled to the territories and thus is routinely subjected to a "special search." It's unpleasant, but she has decided it is better to be honest than to jeopardize her mission and her life dream of fostering peace.

6. Be a Willing Recipient of the Truth from Others

Just as important as telling the truth to others, your goal is also to be a willing recipient of the truth from others. Can you handle the truth? You need to be willing to consider information that may challenge and undermine your core beliefs. You need to be able to take criticism that is truthful and reveals places where you need to grow. When you tell your roommate or partner about a conflict with a coworker, how do you want him to respond? Do you want good counsel—advice about what you did right, what you did wrong, and how you can make amends? Or do you really want to be told that you are blameless and your coworker is 100 percent at fault? Most of the time, most of us want the latter.

Mantras

"May I be free from falsehood."

"Wise people want the truth even more than they want to be right."

Mountain Pose
Tadasana

Are you being straight? Straightness is a sign of honesty. Mountain Pose, the foundational pose of yoga, emphasizes straightness of the whole body. Most of the standing poses in this book begin in this pose.

Build Mountain Pose from the bottom upward.

1 Start with the truth of the floor. Plant your feet firmly on the mat—straight and parallel with each other, hip-width apart. (Now's a great time to ask yourself if you have a truthful understanding of your body. See Explorations question 1 [page 35].) Distribute your weight equally through your feet (forward and back, and side to side).

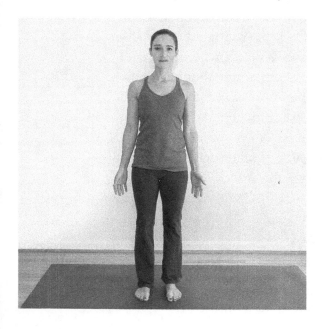

2 Align your knees above your ankles and your hips above your knees. Stack your shoulders on top of your hips and align your ears directly above your shoulders. Straighten your spine. Move your pinky fingers in toward your thighs; palms face forward. Lift the crown of your head slightly, and add an almost imperceptible tilt of your chin downward to your chest.

3 Focus your gaze (*drishti*) straight ahead, at eye level.

Camel Pose
Ustrasana

The emphasis in Camel is often on its heart-opening qualities. Here, I am directing attention to the opening of the throat. According to the chakra system, the throat is the energetic center of our ability to express ourself in healthy and appropriate ways or give voice to our truth.

1 From a kneeling position (knees hip-width apart), lengthen your spine and feel an inward rotation of your thighs (i.e., the muscles in the front of the thighs [the quadriceps] rotate inward to the center line of your body).

2 Curl your toes under or keep the tops of your feet flat on the floor.

3 Bring your hands to the small of your back (fingertips up) and then press your shoulders down your back. Take a deep breath in and lift your sternum up toward the ceiling while your palms press your pelvis and your hips down and forward.

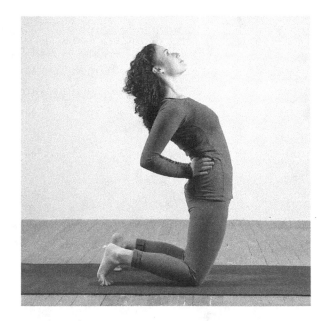

4 Reach the crown of your head as far back as you can without feeling strain on the neck. Maintain length in the front and back of your neck.

Ten-Minute Mindfulness Meditation

A daily ten-minute meditation can help quiet the chattering mind and make space for the truth to reveal itself. It helps to set a timer for ten minutes so that you don't have to keep checking a clock. Begin by finding a comfortable seated position that encourages a straight spine. Rest your hands on your knees or by your thighs. Close your eyes or just soften your gaze. You can spend ten minutes just tuning in to the sensations of sound and touch. Wake up your ears. What do you hear—birds, traffic, air blowing through vents, clocks ticking, conversations in another room? Just make a mental note of what you hear without launching into a story. Or become attuned to the sensation of touch. Can you rekindle your awareness of the feeling of your clothes against your skin or the contact between your body and the chair or the floor?

Another option for a ten-minute meditation is to simply run through the thoughts in your head, as if each thought were a card (as in an old-fashioned Rolodex). You simply name the thought on a card (such as "meeting with boss," "child's report card," "dish-

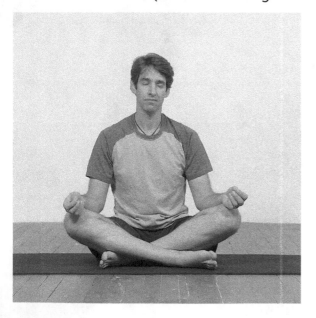

es in sink," "last night's episode of my favorite TV show"), and then mentally flip the card to the next thought. Keep flipping cards while you run through all the thoughts, even as they repeat. Note that our mind is generally limited to no more than five different thoughts at a time. We just keep recycling the same five. As you go through the Rolodex, naming thoughts, you can say "meeting with boss, again," "child's report card, again."

Explorations for Mat, Journal, and Life

1 How well do you know your body? How wide are your hips and shoulders in relation to your yoga mat? What are some examples of when you perceived your body as bigger/smaller, weaker/stronger, more flexible/inflexible than it really is?

2 Recall a time when you told too little of the truth. Recall a time when you told too much of the truth. Which do you tend to do more and why?

3 Do you tend to exaggerate or downplay difficult circumstances, being either a Chicken Little or a Pollyanna?

4 Some people say that most lying is meant to cover up a fear. When you think of a time when you were being dishonest, what were you afraid of? If you keep a "lying" list for a week, are there any patterns in the circumstances that trigger your lying?

5 If you tend to overshare the truth (saying more than necessary), what is your motivation? What are you trying to avoid or attain?

6 Name one or two emotions you are feeling right now (for example, love, joy, hope, gratitude, willingness, humility, anger, sadness, fear, pain, guilt, or shame).

7 How will you practice truth this week? Is there one particular truth you have been avoiding that you can address? Is there one particular relationship that needs a spotlight of truth? Are there patterns to your falsehoods that you can identify and rectify? Are you open to hearing the truth from people you love, people you work with or for, and people you supervise?

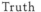

2

Courage

Fear is the cheapest room in the house. I would
like to see you living in better conditions.

Hafiz

The enemy is fear. We think it's hate, but it is fear.

Mahatma Gandhi

Never let your fear decide your fate.

AWOLNATION

Hebrew: *ometz lev* (strong heart)

Sanskrit: *saurya* (sun heart)

There is a famous midrash about the Israelites crossing the Red
Sea. According to the midrash, when the Israelites arrived at
the Red Sea with the Pharaoh's army close behind, the sea did not
immediately part. While some of the Israelites cried in despair,
one young man named Nahshon bravely entered the water. When
the water reached his neck, God was moved to help Moses part
the sea. The name *Nahshon* has come to signify courage—a person who takes risks and leads the way. The story exemplifies an

important feature of this trait. Courage expands possibilities in the face of seemingly limited options. While others felt blocked by the sea in front and the approaching army behind, Nahshon opened an alternative, a path to freedom.

Think of someone acting courageously—a person running into a burning building to save a child, a corporate whistle-blower exposing tainted food products, a political activist standing up to tyranny and corruption. In each case, bravery pushes the person beyond the place of safety, certainty, and comfort. Great acts of

Courage is a state of expansion.

courage may be less dramatic, as when people make midlife career changes, travel overseas alone, or leave abusive relationships. With these examples in mind, we can understand courage as a state of expansion. Courage expands what is possible, broadening the conception we and others hold about what can be accomplished in a given circumstance. When we are acting courageously, we step out of our comfort zone, freeing ourself from the limits imposed on us by our own self and by society.

By contrast, a life lived in fear is a smaller life. Fear is contraction, an involution of us into ourself. Living with fear imperils our spiritual journey in two regards. First, it keeps us from doing what needs to be done, seeing what needs to be seen, and learning what needs to be learned. Fear is an attachment to the status quo, no matter how awful, because it is a known entity. It's clinging to the side of the pool, to the same hopeless job or relationship, to the same patterns and habits of being. In addition, fear is the desire to drop and run, to abandon the current state of things. In yoga, fear can either keep you from lifting your feet off the floor in Headstand or Crow Pose or make you roll up your mat and run out the door. When I am teaching a challenging pose in yoga class, I often remind my students that falling is part of the process of growing. Where would we be if, as children, we weren't willing to risk a few head bonks while learning to walk or do a cartwheel (over and over)? Sure, it's safer to keep both feet on the ground, but it's even safer to crawl. Pushing past fear is the only way to stand tall or fly.

A friend of mine once asked a wise teacher how to find the courage to make big changes in her life, to confront her fears of rejection and find another man to fall in love with and marry. The teacher asked her to think about the cost—all that is being lost—by not changing. Fear of getting hurt emotionally or physically often robs us of more joy than an actual injury. In other words, the pain of loneliness can hurt more than a broken heart. A broken foot heals faster than the regret of never learning how to ski, ride a bike, or rock-climb. A quotation attributed to James Neil Hollingsworth, a beatnik writer and musician, says, "Courage is not the absence of fear, but rather the judgment that something else is more important than fear."

The other impediment fear brings to our spiritual journey is its tendency to eclipse the Divine Presence and feed the illusion of separateness. Consider what Mahatma Gandhi said about the enemy (of goodness and light). Fear of others divides us and feeds our worst impulses. When we are afraid, we are defensive and prone to fall into the traps of discrimination and prejudice. Fear justifies and embellishes our suspicions and distrust of the motives of others. When we presume that someone is a threat to our well-being we cut ourself off from recognizing the divine spark in that person. The more fear, the less light and the darker the perspective.

> Fear is a state of contraction.

Currently in the Middle East there are groups of Israelis and Palestinians joining together to find common ground. Groups like Combatants for Peace and Parents Circle–Families Forum work to bring together the surviving family members from both sides of the conflict to share the commonality of grief and loss. To reach beyond the hate and blame requires us to relinquish fear and embrace courage. To strive for common ground in the midst of such bitterness and divisiveness is to live a brave life of endless expansion.

Play Your Edge

A popular concept in the Western yoga tradition is called "playing the edge." The edge alludes to the borders of your comfort zone. On one side of the comfort zone there is security and ease; on the other there is risk and effort. It is important to remember that living within your comfort zone limits your options. The smaller the comfort zone, the fewer the options. Playing the edge invites you to expand your options by stepping up to the very edge just *beyond* your comfort zone. Your particular edge is as personal as your comfort zone. In a yoga class, your edge could be one of stamina—staying in the pose while your quad muscles burn—or your edge could be going fully upside down in Head- or Hand-stand. In life we have many forms of our edge. Our edge might be speaking in public, making eye contact, eating foods with strange names, flying on a plane, or risking emotional intimacy. No matter what the nature of our edge, when we push ourself to it we expand the radius of our comfort zone and the realm of possibility in our lives; we are living more courageously.

Growing up, I spent my summers at a swim park operated by the local Jewish Community Center. In the days before rampant litigation, the pool offered three diving boards of varying heights: low, medium, and high. Over the years I moved through various stages of hurdles—jumping off the low, forward-diving off the low, backward-diving off the low; jumping off the medium, diving off the medium, backward-diving off the medium; jumping off the high, and so on. Playing your edge is a process. Sometimes your work is just to stay in the edge and breathe, such as when you hold a yoga pose or when you get up to speak in front of a large crowd. Sometimes your work on courage involves taking a leap.

Fear feeds our illusion of separateness.

Playing the edge is a useful exercise in our practice of *Mussar* Yoga, allowing us to get more comfortable with the physical practice of yoga, the spiritual practice of *Mussar*, or the combination of the two. Your comfort zones about yoga, *Mussar*, Judaism, and yourself will surely be challenged. You may feel uneasy with some of the ideas or suggestions you read. You may be asked to confront some elements of your life that you'd prefer to keep unexplored or locked away in a cupboard. Let the concept of playing your edge allow you to engage with the hard work on the *Mussar* Yoga path.

The Contagion of Courage

When you step outside your comfort zone, you give others permission and inspiration to do the same. I see it all the time in *Mussar* classes: Revealing a vulnerability in a group discussion or taking a physical risk in a challenging yoga pose frees others to do the same.

We see the same phenomenon in the actions of the twentieth-century *Mussar* academy leaders, as they lived in the midst of political turmoil and violence. When the stakes were life and death, the *Mussar* movement teachers taught courage by example. Faced with terrible persecution by the Communists to the east and then by the Nazis in the west, the movement's teachers embodied courage and in doing so inspired each other to selfless bravery.

Despite the unfathomable difficulties imposed by wanton violence, curfews, transportation disruptions, and communication censorship, the *Mussar* academies kept in contact with and supported each other. When the leader of the Novarodok movement died during a typhus epidemic, the mourners at his funeral took a vow to "serve with all that remains of our strength, with great fortitude, and stand like a rock in the heart of the seas ... "[1] His heir apparent, desperate to get to Kiev to provide leadership, declared that "one must fear no man."[2] He sought out the brutal communist commander Lev (Leo) Trotsky for assistance, and was then smuggled by troops under Trotsky's command across the conflict's borders. Likewise, when the Communists ordered the closure of one local yeshiva, the dean refused to comply. When the official pointed a rifle at him, the dean "opened his shirt and cried out: 'I am not afraid. Shoot.' Immediately, every student of the yeshiva lined up behind their teacher and did the same." Surprised by the defiance and bravery of the *Mussar* yeshiva, the official backed down and the school remained open.[3]

Courage versus Recklessness

Sometimes fear is legitimate and a good thing. You should probably not walk down a deserted street in the middle of the night in a crime-ridden neighborhood or go skydiving if you are prone to heart attacks. Being reckless or courting trouble are not acts of courage. Courage involves a certain element of wisdom and awareness. It involves discernment.

Likewise, courage doesn't necessarily mean taking action. Sometimes the most courageous act is not acting at all. Our usual temptation in a time of fear or uncertainty is to force certainty in an attempt to control the outcome. The image that comes to mind is soldiers at a checkpoint confronting a person who seems suspicious. Fear prompts an aggressive approach; courage might call for alert restraint.

Courage may be about surrendering expectations and allowing for uncertainty—a cancer patient trying an experimental treatment, for example. One brave friend of mine got onstage in front of a large group of his peers and began to sing a melody he had never sung before. He mispronounced some words and there were a few snickers in the crowd, but before he was finished he had everyone on their feet dancing.

Courage is comfort with uncertainty.

Evaluating risks versus rewards is a valuable exercise, but—and this qualification merits attention—take care not to exaggerate the risks (or the rewards). If you love riding a bike but read in the local paper that someone was hit by a car while riding, don't let fear of an accident keep you off your bicycle, but do be sure to wear a helmet and reflective gear. If you presume that people from different religions, ethnic groups, and nationalities cannot be trusted, then you are letting your smallest and most fearful self win. The middle ground requires an honest evaluation of real risks and rewards with an inclination toward living the most expansive life possible.

Mantras

"Worry is a misuse of imagination."

"Fear no one."

"Fear is the cheapest room in the house."

"Never let your fear decide your fate."

Triangle Pose
Utthita Trikonasana

In this pose, in which we expose our most vulnerable parts—our internal organs and our throat—we feel both our vulnerability and our courage. To choose to be vulnerable is an act of courage. Triangle Pose embodies this contradiction.

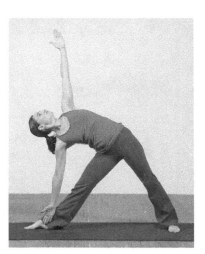

1 From Mountain Pose, step your left leg toward the back of the mat, allowing your feet to be about three feet apart. Keep your right foot pointed forward (twelve o'clock) while your left foot is at an angle so that your left heel is at six o'clock and your left toes are at ten o'clock.

2 Rotate your hips and your shoulders to the left so that your torso is fully facing the left side.

3 Extend your arms to shoulder height. Turn your head and gaze over your right fingertips.

4 Keeping both legs straight, hinge at your right hip and send both hips toward your left leg.

5 Reach with your right arm forward as far as you can. (Imagine reaching over a countertop for a pen while holding on to an old-fashioned corded phone).

6 Then drop your right hand to your shin, a block, or the floor to the outside of your right pinky toe.

7 Reach your left arm high and spread your fingers wide.

8 Refine the pose by stacking your shoulders and aligning them over your rib cage and your right thigh. Drop your tailbone toward your left ankle. Draw your chin off your chest and let all the sides of your neck be long.

Handstand
Adho Mukha Vrksasana

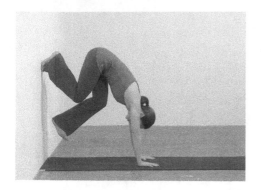

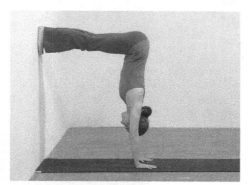

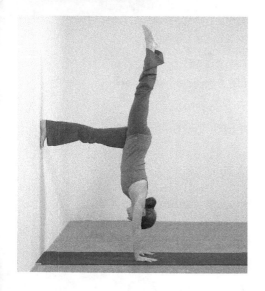

Ready to step out of your comfort zone? This is the mother of all scary poses. Courage requires us to reframe our experience. Think of Handstand as Mountain Pose, but upside down. Being upside down is a way of reframing your whole outlook. Imagine yourself coming up into a straight and strong Handstand.

Note: This pose is not recommended for beginners.

Use a wall at first.

1 Come into Downward Facing Dog with your heels against the wall.

2 Walk both legs up the wall to hip height. Hips are directly above your shoulders and wrists. Your body forms an "L" shape.

3 Lift one leg at a time off the wall. Your gaze or focus (*drishti*) is between your fingertips. Don't be afraid to fall into Wheel Pose (page 70) toward the center of the room. Weigh the real benefits versus the real costs. Handstands build arm strength, teach balance, and convey all the reputed benefits of inversions, including improved circulatory health.

Advanced students can work from the center of the room.

Crow Pose
Bakasana

This is another pose to play your edge if you're a beginner, an advanced student, or in between.

1 Beginning in Mountain Pose in the middle of your mat, toe-heel your feet wider than hip-width apart. Keep your toes slightly turned out.

2 Bend your knees and drop your hips to come into a squat (heels do not need to be on the floor).

3 From the squat, plant your hands on the mat and either squeeze your knees to the outside of your upper arm bones (beginners) or plant your knees directly on your arm bones just below the armpits.

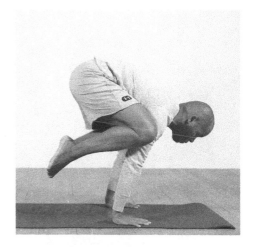

4 Lean your head and upper body forward until you feel the weight of your torso on your arms.

5 Lift one foot and then the other; bring your big toes together while you lift your chest up. Think "up" as you lift through your belly.

6 Beginners can exit the pose by reversing the order, while intermediate and advanced yogis can shoot their legs back into Low Push-up (page 91).

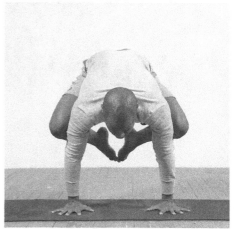

Lion's Breath
Simhasana

Lions are typically thought of as brave animals. You might feel the need to summon some courage when you try this pose in class for the first time; it can feel a little ridiculous at first. Lion's Breath can be practiced from almost any yoga asana; frequently it accompanies Goddess Pose (*Utkata Konasana*), Fish Pose (*Matsyasana*), or Yoga Squat (*Malasana*).

1 Beginners can practice this breathing technique from Easy Seated Pose or in a low kneeling position.

2 To begin Lion's Breath, inhale deeply.

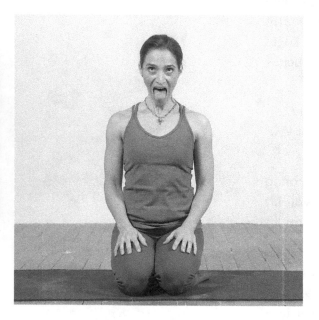

3 Then forcefully exhale through a wide-open mouth, while sticking your tongue far out and downward, rolling your eyes upward, and making a loud roaring sound from the back of your throat.

Explorations for Mat, Journal, and Life

1 When in the past have you exercised braveness on the mat? What was the outcome?

2 Thinking about the past, when in your life have you been notably brave? What risks have you taken? What was the outcome?

3 When was the last time you took a big risk?

4 Identify where and when fear arises in your yoga practice. How do you typically respond to fear in your practice?

5 Where in your life—work, relationships, leisure—is fear holding you back?

6 What would you do if you knew you could not fail?

7 How will you address courage and fear this week? What parts of your upcoming week present opportunities to work on courage? What specifically can you change in your life to act with more bravery? Do you need courage to ask for help? Do you need courage to make a change in your job or a relationship? Do you need to let go of your fear to embark on your life's dream?

3

Humility

The essence of serving God and of all the mitzvot is
to attain the state of humility; to understand that all
your physical and mental power and your essential
being depend on the divine elements within. You
are simply a channel for the divine attributes.

Dov Baer, the Maggid

I am a unique creation, yet my most basic physical substance,
my quarks and my atoms, are identical with those of an
antelope, a redwood, a distant star. I am made of stardust.

Daniel Matt

You are a child of the universe, no less than the
trees and the stars: you have a right to be here.

Max Ehrmann

Hebrew: *anavah*

Sanskrit: *namrata*

On Yom Kippur, a rabbi stops in the middle of the service,
prostrates himself beside the bimah, and cries out, "Oh,
God. Before You, I am nothing!" The cantor is so moved by this

demonstration of pious humility that he immediately throws himself to the floor beside the rabbi and cries, "Oh, God! Before You, I am nothing!" Then Chaim Pitkin, the congregation's president, jumps from his seat, prostrates himself in the aisle, and cries, "Oh God! Before You, I am nothing!" The cantor nudges the rabbi and whispers, "So look who thinks he's nothing."

Humility is the management of ego. The teaching and practicing of *Mussar* Yoga afford me a wide perspective on humility and ego. First and foremost, there's always my ego in the room and I get to see how it plays out when I am the teacher and when I am the student (who is also a teacher). When I'm teaching yoga, it's easy to feel powerful: I say, "Stand up," and a roomful of adults stand up; I say, "Stick out your tongue while standing on one leg and roll your eyes into the back of your head while emitting a loud roaring sound," and, yes, within seconds, a roomful of adults are doing just that. (By contrast, I also teach sociology to college students and when I say, "Read chapter 4 tonight" I probably get 25 percent compliance … at best.) Also, *Mussar* Yoga is a powerful practice, which, on its own, changes lives. People may mistake the message for the messenger. People may come to my *Mussar* Yoga class and leave radically altered. All this may be very heady for any teacher and the dynamic requires us—yoga and *Mussar* teachers— to actively remind ourselves that we're essentially engaged in a messenger service, "a channel for divine attributes," as the Hasidic master Rabbi Dov Ber ben Avraham of Mezeritch, known as the Maggid, called it.

On the other end of things, teaching *Mussar* Yoga offers a clear view of students' egos. The physical poses, *asanas*, are only one small part of the journey to have less suffering in our lives. Sri Pattabhi Jois, a leader of modern yoga, has been quoted as saying that "yoga is an internal practice. The rest is circus."[1] What Jois reminds us is that if the physicality of the practice becomes the end, rather than the means, then the practice is just a performance meant to shore up the ego. I often see students caught up in the circus, chasing down the latest or most complicated, showy pose. And when

I am taking a class, I have to watchfully listen to any voices in my head that say things like "You're a yoga teacher. You should be sitting in full lotus even if your hips are in sharp pain." The ego is a powerful force.

The Challenge of Ego

"If I am not for myself, then who will be for me? And if I am only for myself, then what am I? And if not now, when?" This famous aphorism by Hillel captures the challenge of ego—we must be self-interested but not selfish.

In Jewish tradition, every person is caught between the *yetzer hatov* and the *yetzer hara* (typically translated as the inclination to do good and the inclination to do evil, respectively). A cartoon rendition of an angel and a devil sitting on a character's shoulder is one way to understand the *yetzers*. Rami Shapiro offers another: *yetzer hatov* and *yezter hara* are our selfless and selfish impulses.

A *Mussar* Yoga perspective tweaks this formulation a bit. *Yetzer hatov* may also be interpreted as your spiritual self—the part of you that recognizes that you are made of the same stardust as everything else in the universe and thus your soul is linked to the Divine and the oneness of all creation. *Yetzer hara*, then, is your ego, which emphasizes your uniqueness and separateness from anything else in creation. Although you might think your ego needs to be destroyed—yoga and some traditions of Jewish spirituality hold the annihilation of the self as

> The ego is necessary and problematic.

the highest ideal—the ego is necessary for your day-to-day survival. The ego, in fact, keeps you alive. It allows you to feel a sense of self-worth, which enables you to muster the will to avoid danger, secure food, maintain your health, and build a house.

The ego, then, is simultaneously necessary and problematic from a spiritual perspective. The ego's need to feel different and special competes with the soul's ability to see the oneness of all creation. The same ego that differentiates between you and an approaching truck—and appreciates the difference between the truck's mass, speed, and direction of movement and your human-ness and placement on the road—also differentiates between you and the very smart, talented, and beautiful classmate who is getting all the attention from the teacher and her fellow classmates. This is the same ego that feels superior to others when you notice that your car is nicer, newer, and more expensive than that of any of your neighbors. While the ego is comparing and competing, it is slowly drawing you away from your inner connection to the Divine.

Our work on humility is about creating an appropriate degree of ego—enough to manage the business of living but not so much as to oppress others and drive the presence of God out of existence. When you live with unchecked ego, you doom yourself to discontent and divisiveness. You alienate others with your comparisons and judgments. The ego blinds you to your connection with the world and other living beings, and, on a collective level, ego leads to war, genocide, and ecological destruction.[2]

How do you harness the ego so that its good qualities—those that allow you to feel a sense of honor, self-respect, and appreciation for life—do not trample your soul's ability to connect with the Divine Oneness? You cannot obliterate the ego and survive, yet too much ego can threaten your physical, emotional, and spiritual existence. Cultivating a healthy ego is a challenging undertaking. There are essentially two compatible spiritual approaches to working on humility. One approach is called "balancing ego"; the other is called "managing ego." You can cultivate this trait by doing both simultaneously.

Balancing Ego

The balancing approach views ego on a continuum in which one extreme is complete arrogance and the other is complete meekness or self-effacement. At perfect center lies humility, defined as the proper appraisal of a person's place and space in the world. The balancing approach is a bit of the Goldilocks scenario—neither too much nor too little of the self.

Imagine standing on a balance board, trying to find just the right distribution of weight in the legs. Not too much left or right leg, but an equalizing stance. As you struggle to gain your balance, you rock back and forth—too much right and then, overcompensating, too much left. So it is with our assessments of our self-worth. From self-doubt, we overcompensate with too much arrogance and then shift back to self-doubt. Only when we reach an authentic and loving understanding of who we are and what we can or cannot do can we find the harmony and peace that comes from true humility.

In your efforts to achieve humility, take care not to make any sudden or drastic efforts toward building more confidence or tamping down your conceit. Any move in one direction on the continuum is likely to result in overcorrection on the other side. The trick—and this is not easy at all—is to stay as centered as possible. There are two habits of being that will help you find your center.

Stay centered in your sense of self.

First, stop needing and looking for approval from others or defining your worth by your success. Work hard to cultivate a loving respect for self (take a look at chapter 8, "Equanimity," and chapter 12, "Loving-Kindness and Compassion"). Your sense of self-worth can only come from you, not from anyone else. Remind yourself that you are a holy soul, a piece of the Divine Presence, and so is everyone else.

Second, avoid comparison and competition. The poem "Desiderata" counsels: "If you compare yourself with others, you may become vain and bitter: for always there will be greater and lesser persons than yourself." Start by letting go of competition and comparison on your yoga mat. Find a yoga class without mirrors and pay no attention to what others are doing in their practice. Focus exclusively on your own practice. Take your relinquishment of comparison and competition out the door of the yoga studio into every other facet of your life. Stop caring what car someone else is driving, whether she is skinnier or he has a better-paying job.

Some people can do perfect splits but have messed-up lives, while others can't do perfect splits and have seemingly perfect lives. Let it all go. At the same time, appreciate your own unique gifts and the unique gifts of others.

Neither of these habits is easy to establish. As with all great challenges, start with small steps. You can begin by relinquishing comparison and competition during your yoga practice or during the time you are in synagogue. Or you can practice letting go of a need for approval in the company of family or at work. I have found that the most difficult time to give up these habits is when I am in the company of people who are deeply caught up in their own nets of ego. When someone is trying to compete with me or exert authority in a judgmental way, I have to be extremely mindful not to get thrown off balance. And yet these difficult situations often arise in already high-stress moments when I have the least amount of energy to repel them. When that happens, and I get thrown off balance, the important thing to remember is not to seesaw back and forth on the scales of ego. You can limit the rocking back and forth by working on compassion (chapter 12) with yourself and with the other person.

Here's a famous quotation by spiritual teacher Marianne Williamson from *A Return to Love*. (Notice how she balances both sides of the ego.)

> Our deepest fear is not that we are inadequate. Our deepest fear is that we are powerful beyond measure. It is our light, not our darkness that most frightens us. We ask ourselves, Who am I to be brilliant, gorgeous, talented, fabulous? Actually, who are you not to be? You are a child of God. Your playing small does not serve the world. There is nothing enlightened about shrinking so that other people won't feel insecure around you. We are all meant to shine, as children do. We were born to make manifest the glory of God that is within us. It's not just in some of us; it's in everyone. And as we let our own light shine, we unconsciously give other people

permission to do the same. As we are liberated from our own fear, our presence automatically liberates others.[3]

Managing Ego

The other technique for dealing with ego involves size management. Specifically, this tactic, which is part of both yoga and mystical forms of *Mussar*, aims to make the ego as small as possible. In this approach, we can think of the ego as a balloon and our work involves shrinking or deflating it.

The smaller the space that the ego occupies, the closer we come to the Divine Presence, as if the expansion of the ego balloon pushes God further away from our soul. Mystics may dream of the complete and permanent destruction of the ego, but most of us achieve only moments—sometimes just seconds—when we feel a deep connection to the Divine and all of creation. Reaching out and caring about others deflates the ego. When someone else's success means the same to us as our own, our identification and attachment to self weakens or disappears. We loosen the grip on our bounded sense of self, our I-ness. Then, our sense of self merges with the Divine Presence.

In Kabbalah, there is a concept called *tzimtzum*. *Tzimtzum* refers to the contraction of the Divine Presence in the world in order to make space for the rest of creation. In the Foreword to *Saying No and Letting Go*, Naomi Levy writes about personal *tzimtzum* that can be applied to ego management. "Through contraction we make room—for others, for God, for miracles, and for surprise. By contracting we actually grow. We learn to hear what others are really trying to say to us, we learn to hear the voice of our own souls, and we learn to hear the voice of God calling out to us."[4]

Even though managing the size of the ego sounds heady and impossibly difficult, there are very easy and concrete steps we can take to diminish the power of the ego. In *A New Earth*, spiritual innovator Eckhart Tolle observes that certain behaviors inflate the ego. The four types of behaviors to avoid are:

Complaint

Resentment

Reactivity

Grievance

Complaint—that is, identifying something wrong with other people, situations, and organizations—pumps up the ego. When the ego is distracted by external fault-finding, it seeks relief from its own internal criticism. The ego affirms its superiority by finding problems with other people and situations.

Resentment, says Tolle, dovetails with complaint. It's the emotion (anger or indignation) that accompanies complaint. It is possible to find fault without generating resentment. You can ask your spouse for more help in the house without coming from a place of anger, for example.

Reactivity is the residual emotional charge you get from feeling resentment. Some people live their lives feeling angry because anger energizes and motivates them. They tend to hold on to grievances for decades. We all know folks who can't forget a slight made against them twenty years ago.

Grievances can span generations and create legacies of division and discord, like the ongoing feud between the Hatfields and the McCoys.

Along with avoiding those four behaviors, we can manage our ego by seeking a sense of commonality and connectivity. When your ego identifies a flaw in another person, make it your humility practice to find a similar flaw within yourself and compassionately embrace our collective flawed existence. When you're stuck in traffic, and your ego identifies the *other* cars on the road as the problem, consider it a humbling reminder that, to those other drivers, you and your car are the problem. And when your ego is threatened by someone else's success, let your *Mussar* Yoga practice be to share in that person's success. Avoid seeing success as a zero-sum game—that

Contract your ego to make room for others.

someone else's success diminishes the worth and value of you and your work in any way.

Following are three yoga postures for our *Mussar* work to balance and manage the ego. In your home practice or class this week, keep the lessons of this *Mussar* trait in your consciousness. Overall, consider the following observation, by B. K. S. Iyengar, about the appearance of ego in any endeavor: "The ego is an unrelenting taskmaster. It does not know that one must balance activity and passivity in the *asana*, exertion and relaxation."[5] This leads to injury. Your first *Mussar* work in any pose is to take the ego out of the practice by letting go of attachment to outcome rather than process. And, in every pose, let breath be the reminder of your humility.

Mantras

"I'm enough."

"We are all made of stardust—stars in the sky and dust on the ground."

"Who are you not to be?"

Warrior I
Virabhadrasana I

This stance invites a sense of confidence and purposeful strength, yet at the same time its challenging alignment keeps us humble. Warrior I is also a great pose to explore the "unrelenting taskmaster" of ego. Find the balance of activity and passivity—toes relax while feet engage, shoulder blades draw in while the tops of the shoulders soften and drop, and eyes are steady and focused while the jaw unclenches.

1 Starting in Mountain Pose, exhale and step your left foot to the back of the mat. Angle your left foot by keeping your left heel at six o'clock and pointing your left toes to ten o'clock.

2 Bend your front leg until your knee is right above your ankle. Your back leg remains straight. Square your hips by pulling your left hip forward and drawing your right hip back. Extend your arms overhead.

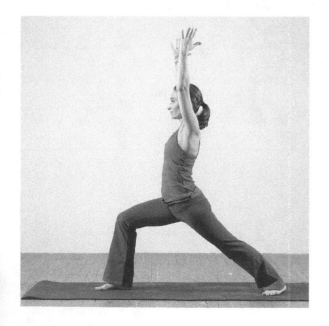

3 Refine the pose by dropping your shoulders down your back while pulling your shoulder blades together. Anchor your left pinky toe into the mat and lift up the inner arch of your foot.

4 Move into Humble Warrior (see below) before you repeat on the left.

Humble Warrior
Baddha Virabhadrasana

Practicing Humble Warrior increases both quadriceps strength and shoulder flexibility. The combination is a good reminder that humility requires us to be resilient and yet willing to bend and be flexible when appropriate.

1 From Warrior I on the right, reach your hands behind your back and interlace your fingers.

2 On an inhale, lift your sternum upward and then, as you exhale, drop your chest forward. Your rib cage can hover over your front thigh (as pictured) or you can drop lower and ease your chest over the big toe side of your right foot. Keep your spine and neck elongated.

3 Lift your arms off your back as high and forward as they can go.

4 Practice this pose on both sides.

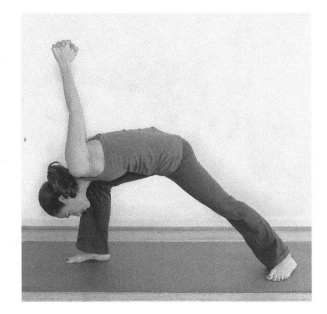

Half Moon
Ardha Chandrasana

Half Moon is the perfect pose to practice humility and check the ego. It's a challenging pose and, once you learn it, it seems to invite a sense of hubris. The moment, though, that your ego is engaged, you lose your balance and fall.

1 From Mountain Pose, step your left leg to the back of your mat and angle your left foot so that your left heel is at six o'clock and your toes are at twelve o'clock. Drop your right hand at a slight diagonal toward your right pinky toe and then slowly lift your left leg to hip height.

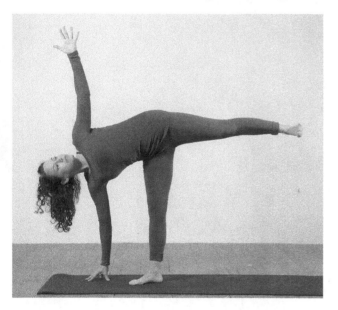

2 Rotate your left hip on top of your right and extend your left arm up to the ceiling, so that your hips and shoulders are vertically stacked.

3 Repeat on the right side.

Headstand
Sirsasana

Anything that puts your head (ego) below the rest of the body is a good way to recalibrate your sense of self. And there's nothing like falling and landing belly side up again and again to keep you humble. Again, there's nothing like coming up into an inversion, holding it, feeling a sense of pride well up, and then falling out of it, yet again, to keep your ego in check.

Try your first Headstands against a wall until you get over the initial fear and uncertainty.

1 Keeping your arms shoulder-width apart, from Downward Facing Dog drop onto your forearms (elbows at shoulder-width) and interlace your fingers (your hands should be two to three inches from the wall).

2 Drawing your shoulder blades together, walk your feet toward your hands until your hips are directly above your shoulders.

3 Lower the crown of your head onto the mat, allowing your hands to cradle the back of your head. Keep drawing your shoulder blades together to support your neck.

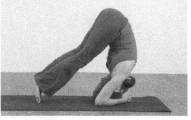

4 Pull one knee to your chest and, when you feel steady and supported enough, lift your other knee to your chest. Over time, begin to raise both legs above your head.

5 Stay in the pose for several rounds of breath, working your way to staying in the Headstand for three to five minutes.

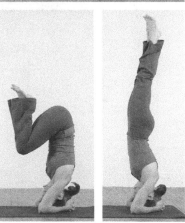

Note: This pose is *not* for people with neck injuries or neck weakness. See other inversion restrictions noted on page 17. The safest way to practice any forward inversion is under the guidance of a trained instructor.

Explorations for Mat, Journal, and Life

1. How big a role does ego play in your practice? How often do you attempt or fully practice poses that are too demanding for your body at the moment, but that feed your ego?

2. What are ways you can let go of the performance element of the practice and just allow your awareness of breath (*prana*) to deepen?

3. How do the conditions for ego—complaint, comparison, resentment, and grievance—show up in your practice? How do they show up in your life?

4. What does the world look like when you see it through the lens of oneness? What do your relationships with others look like when viewed this way?

5. What are proactive ways you can take care of yourself during practice? (For example, remembering to breathe deeply and backing off any poses that take you out of sweet, rhythmic breathing.)

6. What is your homework for cultivating humility this week? Where in your life are you playing too small, acting too humble? Where in your life are you feeding your ego with comparison, resentments, and grievances? Is there a particular relationship or circumstance that triggers ego challenges for you? Can you keep a daily journal and list the times that your ego was too small or too big?

4

Order

A season is set for everything, a time for
every experience under heaven.

Ecclesiastes 3:1

Our body is the home of our spirit. It is the means by
which we enact our beliefs. Therefore, the maintenance
of the body is a spiritual duty, an act of love not
only toward ourselves but toward all humanity.

Rolf Gates

Invention, it must be humbly admitted, does not
consist in creating out of void, but out of chaos.

Mary Shelley

Hebrew: *seder*

Sanskrit: *saucha*

At my first brief introduction session to *Mussar*, we broke out
into small groups to work on particular traits. A friend of mine
chose order and her group work generated an "aha" moment. She

realized that getting more organized was an easy way to gain more inner peace. The fix was simple. By reducing the turmoil from the daily frantic scrambling for lost car keys or a missing purse, she could have more moments of calmness. She returned from the workshop and spent the next few weeks cleaning out rooms, placing new hooks on the walls for keys and coats, and installing new bins for recycling and Goodwill giveaways. As she cleared away the clutter, she made space for greater efficiency and productivity. She felt less stressed about work and her relationship with her family, and her feelings about her house and even her life improved. She observed that she had always considered the disorder in her house "no big deal," but in retrospect it was a really big deal, indeed.

As Ecclesiastics proclaims, everything has a rightful place in both time and space. When our lives are in proper order, our energy flows more smoothly. Emotions, possessions, behaviors, relationships, school, work, and leisure all fare much better when they are in a state of order.

Order applies to physical things in space, time, and energy.

Typically when we think of order, we think of physical order—the placement of things—in physical space. In simple terms, we think about what objects go in what physical space. That is, the pile of paper goes in the recycling bin or a file cabinet; the dirty dishes go in the sink or, better still, in the dishwasher. This type of physical ordering is important. As my friend learned, we do profit from better organization of our belongings. When we tidy up our physical world, we create a sense of discipline for ourself and a degree of efficiency in our lives.

Order applies to other dimensions of living as well. We can order time and activities. There is an optimal time in the day for eating, sleeping, working, and socializing. We need to engage in those activities in the right amount at the appropriate times in a twenty-four-hour cycle. Ordering time can be as challenging as organizing space. There are many things that vie for our attention and time. I've been told that a certain rabbi would ask the office staff to block off a few hours on his weekly calendar for study and writing. He even instructed them to inform callers that he was in a meeting, saying it was true because "I am in a meeting with myself." By contrast, I've sat down to lunch with friends who spent more time answering their cell phones than they did talking with me.

There's a saying in yoga: "Where the mind goes, energy flows." Even our thoughts need ordering. Maybe you've been giving too much thought to work and not your family, or too much energy to the logical side of your brain and not enough to the wellsprings of art and creativity in your life. In the *Mussar* classic *Chesbon ha-Nefesh*, Rabbi Mendel upbraided people who walk through the marketplace with their minds elsewhere, tripping over objects, bumping into others, causing mayhem, and embarrassing themselves. The work of ordering, carving out time and space, asks us to clean out, pull apart, and then examine all the structures and habits of our lives.

Creating Order Is Spiritual Work

Cleaning out the basement or deleting old e-mails may feel, at best, mundane or, at worse, like drudgery, but the process has a deeply spiritual context. Creating order is about making space; it is an act of creation. Genesis is an account of order created from chaos, making space for the creation of the world as we know it. From the unformed void, God separated light from dark, and earth and water from sky. From that ordering the Infinite Presence also created celestial bodies of the sky and earthly bodies, both animal and human. Fashioning order from chaos in our own lives is spiritual work in the sense that we are replicating the work of God. The precise ordering of worship services and the Passover seder (which literally translates as "order") emphasize the importance of this trait in our spiritual curriculum.

Typically the yogic discipline of *saucha* finds expression through the idea of personal or bodily cleanliness. House cleaning and cleansing of the body are forms of order—moving dirt and grime to their proper location or refraining from eating dirty or unhealthy foods to keep the inside of the bodily temple pure.

Saucha requires that we arrive on our yoga mat in a state of cleanliness—having bathed and wearing clean clothing. Most spiritual traditions require some form of cleansing as a holy act to prepare to encounter the purity of the Sacred. Religious rituals of purification include washing hands or whole body immersion in water (such as the *mikveh*), or the tidying or cleaning of quarters or belongings before an important occasion (such as cleaning the house before Passover).

The Beauty of Chaos

In Genesis, chaos (*tohu* in Hebrew) precedes creation. Not only is there spiritual meaning in the work of order, but there is also spiritual value in chaos. Rabbi David Cooper, a leading contemporary teacher of mystical Judaism, teaches that, according to Kabbalah, the chaos that preceded the creation of the world was the "breaking of the vessels." (These vessels had contained the various emanations of God.) The expression *tikkun olam* (repair of the world), in essence, refers to the work of ordering—bringing back together the various emanations of God.

The value of chaos as a prompt for creation means that there's a time and space for mess. Chaos is fertile ground for breaking the chains of habit and finding new worlds and new ways of living. Chaos breaks down entrenched patterns and habits. Too little chaos is as dangerous as too much. The right amount of chaos frees us from the status quo. Without a tolerance for some chaos, we will be stuck and trapped in old systems of order that don't serve us anymore. The paradox of order is that often, in the cleaning process, things get messier before they get cleaner. When we're cleaning out a closet, all the chaos on the inside has to first make its way out. We pull out well-worn shoes, socks, or gloves with missing mates, plus half-filled boxes with items whose worth is long forgotten. The mess goes from contained to uncontained as the area around the closet is strewn with the closet debris. In fact, the greater the mess we create in the process of making order, the deeper and more complete our new ordering can be. We may pull out all the junk in the closet, but until we also drag out the boxes of stuff and sort through them, the available space in our closet will not be maximized.

Babies have a primitive instinct called the Moro reflex. When an infant feels a loss of support, a sense of falling, her arms instinctively extend and then draw in (hug and grip). By the time we are four or five months old, we've lost that particular reflex, but our fear of falling—especially emotionally—ingrains in us a lifetime pattern of grasping and gripping on to some real or, more likely illusory, semblance of stability.

One of the primary purposes of taking a hot power yoga class is to throw our minds and bodies into chaos in order to get us to loosen our grip on life and invite more freedom, spontaneity, and creativity. When we have too much order, we lose creative spontaneity. In his workshops, power yogi Rolf Gates instructs his students to loosen the grip they hold on life. A *vinyasa* flow—a series of yoga poses with coordinated breathing—moves very quickly and pushes people physically until they loosen that grip, the clenching, controlling reflex. Only when we become too exhausted to hold on to the old order do we let go and allow for chaos and re-ordering. We need to release our grip on the old, haul everything out into the light, and let a new and improved order emerge.

There is time and space for chaos and dirt.

One morning in yoga class I was helping my students drop back into Wheel Pose after flipping their Downward Facing Dog. At first the move seems very complicated, as it involves shifting your weight into your legs and spinning your bottom fingers from pointing forward to back. One of my students exclaimed, "My mind feels like one big mess." "Perfect," I responded, "because mess precedes order. No mess, no order."

Not only can our grasping for order keep us from reaping the fruits of chaos, but also sometimes an overattachment to order thinly masks our need for control. The relationship between anxiety and control is well known. In the name of order, we may be demanding control and avoiding fear. One woman's mother used to get completely bent out of shape when houseguests came to visit. She would find a dish in the sink or toys on the floor and, instead of recognizing the temporary nature of the disorder, she would insist that all the kids (and adults) conform to her rules of order. Sociologists have noted that the modern interest in landscaping—the ordering of nature itself, not for food but for the illusion of control—reflects other modern desires for control and order.[1] These days we sometimes become rigid in our demands about the

> An unmoderated demand for order can mask an unrelenting need for security and control.

food we eat, insisting on the presence or absence of particular ingredients. Sometimes the motivation is medical, but oftentimes there is an unexamined anxiety and desire for control, as if we could live for an eternity if we ate only the correct whole grains, free-range eggs, organically grown tomatoes, and heirloom blueberries. At the extreme of ordering is a mental condition called obsessive-compulsive disorder (OCD). OCD is a type of anxiety disorder in which people attempt to control their fears and their environment through elaborate rules and rituals of ordering—handwashing, door locking (and unlocking), or arranging books, records, or other possessions in alphabetical order.

When we work on the trait of order, we must be especially mindful of our tendencies to either avoid or cede control to chaos. Too much of either one is problematic, yet in proper balance an ordered life (open to periodic chaos) is a productive life and allows us to make ourself in the image of the Divine.

Mantras

"Everything has a place in time and space."

"Make space for new possibilities."

"No mess, no order."

Side Plank
Vasisthasana

Every time I teach this pose, I see students struggle to find their balance because they don't believe that sometimes things have to get messier before they get in order. The challenge of Side Plank involves the balancing of weight with the hips and the head. In this pose the hips must press forward while the head draws backward, but most students get nervous with the instability of the pose when they press their hips forward. Instead of allowing themselves to fall a few times while they figure out the best alignment, they choose to stick with the safety of hips back and head forward. Finding the proper alignment in this pose reminds us that, at first, putting things together may feel a lot like taking things apart.

1 If you're a beginner, from Downward Facing Dog you can drop your right knee to the center of the mat and roll onto the big toe side of your left foot (left heel falls to the right). Intermediate and advanced students can come into Plank Pose and spin both heels to the right, stacking the inner edges of the feet—big toe touching big toe.

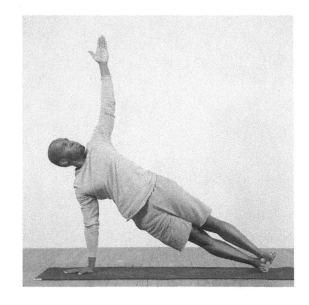

2 Lift your left arm upward and gaze at your left thumb.

3 Pike up your hips.

4 Press your hip bones forward and draw your head back— aligning your right ear over your right hand. Repeat on the left side.

Flipped Dog, with Variation
Camatkarasana

You need to put up with a fair amount of chaos in this pose before you learn the correct timing and weight distribution.

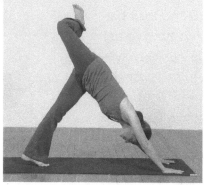

1 Begin in Downward Facing Dog. Extend your right leg behind you. Lift it as high as you can, allowing for your right hip to fully rotate above your left.

2 Bend your right knee and flex your right foot.

3 Lift your left heel off the mat, coming onto your left toes.

4 Lift your right hand off the mat and let your right foot drop behind you.

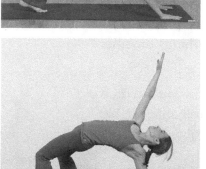

5 Bring both feet flat on the mat, hip-width apart.

6 Reach your right arm up and then, with your thumb as your focus (*drishti*), begin to reach your right hand over your head toward the floor.

7 If you want to drop into a Full Wheel (*Urdhva Dhanurasana*) from step 6, shift your weight into your feet and begin to bend your left elbow. This maneuver also requires you to turn the position of your bottom hand so that your fingers point toward your feet.

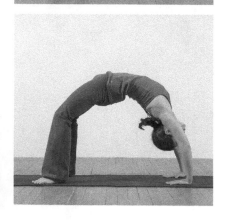

8 Come out of the pose by following in reverse the steps you took to come into it. Repeat on the other side.

Alternate Nostril Breathing
Nadi Sodhana

Alternate Nostril Breathing (ANB) is a form of *pranayama*, a practice of managing our vital life force (called *prana* in Sanskrit).[2] I generally sequence this *pranayama* exercise right before Corpse Pose (*Savasana*) (see page 105). ANB has a calming effect because it pulls our focus to a specific order of breathing.

ANB uses the right thumb and the right ring and pinky fingers. (The index and middle finger can either rest on the third eye or press into the palm.)

1 To begin, find a comfortable position, such as Easy Pose, and close your eyes.

2 Place your right thumb on your right nostril.

3 Take a full, deep breath through your left nostril.

4 Then place your right ring and pinky fingers on your left nostril. Hold your breath in for a moment.

5 Release your thumb from your right nostril and exhale fully on the left side.

6 Inhale deeply through the right nostril before closing it off with your right thumb. Hold your breath in for a moment.

7 Release your ring and pinky fingers on the left, and exhale fully through the left nostril.

8 Keep repeating this sequence for multiple rounds of breath. On the last round, end with an exhalation on the right side and then release your hands to your lap. Sit quietly and feel the full effects of ordered breath.

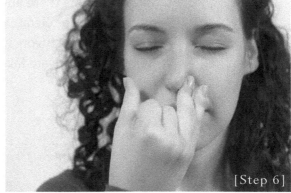

[Step 6]

Explorations for Mat, Journal, and Life

1 How does your yoga practice mirror the order or disorder of the rest of your life?

2 How much attention do you pay to the alignment of your poses—too much or not enough? Where in your practice do you sacrifice joy and freedom for proper alignment, and where do you set yourself up for injury by ignoring proper alignment?

3 What moments in your daily life could benefit from using breathing techniques that help you put aside your thoughts and create a space for being in the present moment?

4 How much time do you spend cleaning or organizing instead of enjoying life? How much time do you spend looking for missing objects, such as keys, glasses, or papers?

5 How does your level of organization and order reflect or respond to your need to have control in your life?

6 How can you find a spiritual component to your practice of order this week? What parts of your life would benefit most from more order? Are there any areas where you are too controlling and unwilling to tolerate chaos? Are there any routines or patterns of living that work adequately, but could be dramatically improved if they were taken apart and reassembled differently?

5

Nonjudgment

Out beyond ideas of wrong doing and right
doing, there is a field. I'll meet you there.

Rumi

Oneness is the norm, the standard and the goal. If in the
afterglow of a religious insight we can see a way to gather
up our scattered lives, to unite what lies in strife—we know
it is a guidepost on His way ... If a thought generates pride,
separation from other people's suffering, unawareness of the
dangers of evil—we know it is a deviation from His way.

Abraham Joshua Heschel

Hebrew: *kavod*

Sanskrit: *ahimsa*

Discernment is part of human nature. Our survival depends on
determining friend or foe, safe or dangerous, kind or cruel.
Beyond that, the arts and culture exist because we develop discernment for varying levels of what is true, good, and beautiful.
Unfortunately for most of us, though, our discernment extends

well beyond survival, arts, and culture. We spend a lot of our lives judging other people in terms of how they act, what they wear, who they associate with, and what they own.

In a *Mussar* group I facilitated, one participant admitted that practicing nonjudgment during the Jewish High Holy Days would be difficult because so many of her encounters with friends and family at the synagogue involved judgment of other people—what so-and-so was wearing, what her kids were wearing, what her husband said ... the list goes on. (Did you just catch yourself judging the judgers?) When we take time for awareness of judgment, we may be surprised by how much it consumes our time and attention.

Our addiction to judgment reflects the degree to which we are slaves to our ego. Judgment is a way of protecting and empowering our ego. Humility and nonjudgment are inextricably linked. Tara Brach, founder of the Insight Meditation Center of Washington (D.C.), wrote: "The more inadequate we feel, the more uncomfortable it is to admit our faults. Blaming others temporarily relieves us from the weight of failure."[1] When we feel rotten about ourself and our accomplishments, we turn our blistering critical eye from ourself to others. During a yoga workshop led by Live Love Teach cofounder Philip Urso, he asked us to think of

Ego and judgment are inextricably linked.

someone in our lives who is a "jerk." He asked us to summon the "jerk's" name and image into our minds and then to make a mental list of all the things he does that make him a jerk. Finally, Urso posed this question, "Have you ever done any of the same things as the jerk?" The answer, of course, is yes. We've all done all those things. His point is that we project our condemnation of ourself onto others. What we see and despise in others we hold within us.

Yoga maven Judith Lasater links nonjudgment with the yogic practice of *ahimsa* (nonviolence).[2] Judgment is a form of violence. It is a violence we perpetrate on ourself and on the people around us. Ironically, those of us who feel strongly about peace in our cities, in our country, and around the world may exercise the most judgmental violence upon ourselves and the people we love.

When we judge, we also pull ourself away from oneness and union with the Divine. When we attack ourself, we fail to see the divinity within us, and when we attack others we lose sight of the divinity within all creation. Judgment then helps create and sustain an illusion of separateness and difference on which the ego and conflict feed.

One of the first steps to minimizing our judgmental tendencies is to simply become aware of when they arise. Judgment easily becomes habit and the backdrop to internal and external chatter. Figure out the tendencies or patterns of your criticism. Keep track of when and what you judge. Ask yourself whether you are bothered most by what others do or by what others say. Determine whether you critique superficial things, such as appearances and material possessions, or deeper issues that concern values and morals. It is particularly helpful to determine the external factors (that is, social circumstances) and internal conditions (that is, your emotional state) that are most likely to spawn judgment. Gain insight into how often you are critical of your coworkers, sales clerks, other parents in your child's playgroup, other drivers when you're in the car, or other people in your neighborhood or social groups.

Honoring Others, Honoring Ourself

When we stop judging we can begin to see more clearly the Divine in us and in others. Both yoga and Judaism regard the soul as a piece of the Universal Divine within us. In yoga the divine soul is called *jivatman* (the Universal Divine is *atman*). The Hebrew word for soul is *neshama*, a pure, incorruptible connection to Divine Oneness. Many yoga classes end with the invocation of the Sanskrit word *namaste*, which translates as "the divine light in me honors the divine light in you." The ability to recognize a piece of the Divine in someone else allows me to more fully feel the divinity within myself. *Honor* means to recognize the Divine Presence in another, to see the intrinsic value and worth in another being.

When we honor others, we enter into the presence of God. In a lecture to our Baltimore Wexner Heritage group, Rabbi Lawrence

A. Hoffman expressed the idea that our meaningful interactions with other people can be a way of experiencing God.[3] What I think Rabbi Hoffman means is that any time we establish a real connection with others, we have transcended our ego and moved into the space of Divine Oneness.

There are essentially two good ways to honor people in your midst, and they are both very simple. We honor people when we truly *see* them and they feel they have been seen. There's a big difference between seeing someone and really seeing someone. The latter is about making eye contact and giving full attention to the person or people in front of you. When you look your coworker, the store clerk, the waiter, the janitor, the toll collector on the highway, the barista, or the hotel maid in the eye, you acknowledge her presence, his humanity, her worth. You affirm that each one is not just another soulless provider of service, like a telephone, a television, or a vending machine. Simply and honestly seeing a person and letting her know that she has been seen can transform everyday encounters into meaningful interactions that invite the presence of God. Making eye contact in every encounter can radically transform your relationships and deepen your spirituality.

> We honor people when we truly see and hear them.

Honor is not only connected to the practice of seeing the other, but to listening, too. Just like seeing, there is hearing and then there is really hearing, which is listening. Making someone feel heard is not easy when you're paying a toll on the Pennsylvania Turnpike, although there's a famous story in my family about one toll collector yelling to another, "Brenda made the honor roll." (My aunt extended her congratulations to Brenda's mother.) But really listening to someone means being willing to stop, hear her words, and consider her viewpoint. Listening goes beyond what we hear with our ears; it means thoughtfully considering whatever another person is trying to communicate to us. In that vein, listening with honor means we should be careful before we hit SEND on our e-mails and texts. Just the other day, my husband read an e-mail from a colleague at work. At first glance the wording seemed confrontational, but after my husband reread the e-mail, he realized that the intent was, in fact, rather deferential. The difference between hearing confrontation (and escalation) and deference is profound. Only when we take time to hear what another is really saying do we forge true connection and gain the ability to move away from judgment.

Cultivating the discipline of a mindful gaze or concentration on sound is important. Yoga teaches that where you look in a pose— that is, your focus (*drishti*)—affects your practice and the quality of your action. It's obvious, for example, when someone is taking a picture of you, that the effect if you look into the camera is different than if you look down at the floor. On a metaphorical level, if you are always looking for what is wrong, you will only ever see a very flawed world. Rabbi Edward Feinstein, in his book *Tough Questions Jews Ask: Teacher's Guide*, recounts a fable about Berel and Shmerel who left Egypt with Moses. "As slaves these two had grown so accustomed to looking down at the ground they could no longer lift their eyes." At the crossing at the Red Sea, all they could see was mud, at Mount Sinai, all they could hear was a voice shouting commands, and as they entered the Promised Land, all they could feel was their feet hurting. Because they could not raise their focus, the two could not see that the conditions of freedom were superior to those of slavery. And so they returned to Egypt, where they remained slaves.[4]

In addition, yoga suggests that we also train ourself to listen. Tuning in to sound enhances our ability to be present. By cultivating a *drishti* of breath, we promote our capacity to listen to others without letting our minds wander. It is also helpful to train ourself to listen without formulating our next response. The most central and important prayer in all of Judaism is the *Shema*:

Shema, Yisrael, Adonai Eloheinu, Adonai echad.

Hear, O Israel, the Eternal is our God, the Eternal is One! (Deuteronomy 6:4)

Shema means "listen." The *Shema* commands us to listen as a means of honoring the Divine Presence that exists both outside all of us and within each of us.

Finding Balance

There are, of course, some behaviors and actions that demand judgment—those that hurt other people in a direct and purposeful way. A father's decision to buy his daughter a brand-new BMW for her sixteenth birthday does not really hurt anyone. Even though I can argue that it makes my job as a parent that much more difficult, I should not judge the values and decisions of others. On the other hand, a parent who provides or allows underage drinking at her house, risking the lives of teenagers and other drivers on the road, is deserving of judgment followed by action (contacting other parents, school authorities, or the police).

Nonjudgment does not mean that we accept all behaviors. We can and should distinguish between what is noble and what is not. But we should be careful in our judgments. The great twentieth-century Jewish theologian and philosopher Abraham Joshua Heschel advised, "If a thought generates pride, separation from other people's suffering, unawareness of the dangers of evil—we know it is a deviation from His way." When our discernments serve our ego, when they reinforce the idea that we are somehow better than others, we are shutting off access to God.

Mantras

"Namaste."

"The divine light in me honors the divine light in you."

"Shema."

Eagle Pose
Garudasana

In this pose, imagine an eagle perched on the top of a tree, surveying the world around him. In this moment he is the picture of discernment, scanning the landscape for what is food and what is danger. In Eagle Pose, we want to acknowledge the power and importance of discernment. Balancing poses often bring out frustration and self-judgment. When a balance goes well, we feel good about ourself and our practice. But when we struggle with balancing, we start to form harsh judgments about ourself and our practice.

Note that your goal is to remove *all* judgment from any pose. Aim to discern whether on a given day you found the pose challenging or easy, but leave the labels of *good* and *bad* behind.

1 Modify your Mountain Pose by bringing your feet together until your big toes touch and your heels are a smidgen apart.

2 Bend both knees and then lift your right knee toward your chest.

3 Wrap your right thigh tightly around your left thigh and squeeze both thighs together until you can, perhaps, tuck your right foot behind your left calf muscle.

4 Extend your arms straight in front of you, shoulder-height, and then cross your right arm beneath your left so that your arms meet at the elbows.

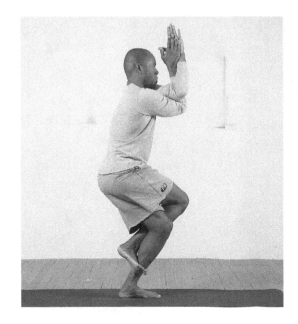

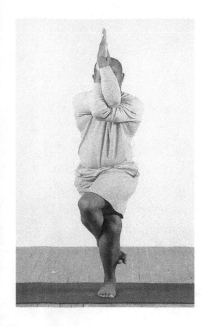

5 Bend both elbows and lift your fingertips skyward, bringing either the back of your hands together or your palms together.

6 Lift your elbows off your chest and focus straight ahead, at eye level.

7 Repeat on the left side, being mindful to reverse your arms. When your left leg is wrapped on top of your right (left leg dominant), your left arm will drop below your right arm (left arm nondominant).

Warrior III
Virabradrasana III

In a crowded class, you might find someone else's foot in your face while doing Warrior III. It may even connect with your chin or nose. When this happens to me, it can bring up a lot of judgment! I might come out of my pose to study how far back on his mat the guy in front of me is standing. "Listen, buddy," I want to shout, "you're way too tall to be taking this pose from the middle of your mat. You must be very selfish." When people get in our space, we start to feel judgmental about their character. Or someone around you might be wobbly and throw you off your balance. Use this pose to gain awareness of your judgment of others.

1 You can come into Warrior III from Mountain Pose by simply extending your left leg behind and upward.

2 Hips are hinged and 90 degrees from your right leg—drop your left hip to meet the height of your right hip.

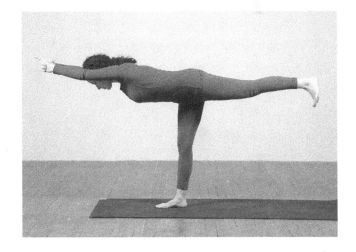

3 Warrior III looks like a capital "T." Stretch your arms forward to be in line with your ears.

4 Repeat the pose on the left side with the right leg extended.

Seated Forward Bend
Paschimottanasana

Sometimes this *asana* is referred to as East-West Pose. This name gives you the sensation of a deep stretch. Think of this pose as a work in progress. You can spend a lot of time judging yourself or others in this pose. If your nose touches your knees, good for you, but most of us have a lot of blue sky between our chest and our thighs. Being in a place of nonjudgment is a place of peace. Be okay with where you are. Be at peace.

1 Begin from Easy Pose and then uncross your legs and extend them straight forward.

2 To tilt the pelvic "bowl" forward, reach your right hand behind and underneath your right buttock and pull your "hip flesh" straight back. Do the same on the left and you should feel more forward momentum from your pelvic region.

3 Keep your feet and toes active and pointing straight up. Pull the pinky toe sides of your feet back toward you while pressing the big toe sides forward and away from you.

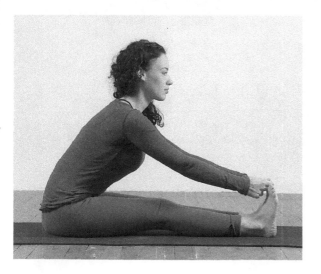

4 Extend your arms overhead and fold forward.

5 Your lower back should remain as flat as possible, while allowing for a slight and natural curve of your midsection. Don't overly round the back in an effort to touch your toes or pull your nose to your knees.

Explorations for Mat, Journal, and Life

1 What kinds of judgment do you hold about your own body? What judgments do you hold about your appearance, your physical strength or flexibility, your performance on the mat during a given practice?

2 What other judgments come up during a yoga class? Do you judge the teacher—how she teaches, how she looks, what music she plays, what sequences she offers? Do you judge other people in the class—their practice, their appearance, their "yoga-ness"?

3 What connections can you make between your own insecurities and your judgment of others?

4 What can you do when you are around other people who are judging others in an unfair, ego-driven manner?

5 How will you implement nonjudgment this week? Can you catch yourself passing judgment on others, noticing any patterns in terms of when, what, why, who, and where you tend to judge? Or is your work this week to focus on finding ways to honor other people? Who needs you to see or hear them more? Are there family, friends, acquaintances, or strangers to whom you can give honor?

6

Zeal

Saw a little girl touch a big bug and shout, "I conquered
my fear! YES!" and calmly walk away. I was inspired.

Nathan Fillion

Enthusiasm is the mother of effort, and without
it nothing great was ever achieved.

Ralph Waldo Emerson

Hebrew: *zerizut*

Sanskrit: *tapas*

One day in college, my best friend noted in passing that while
I enthusiastically initiated grand projects, my track record for
completion was fairly poor. His comment landed heavily; I had
never really considered my tendency to slack off at the end. But I
conceded that his observation was spot-on and it got me to focus
on an important skill—learning to stay in the fire from start to finish.

Zeal refers to the energy we bring to our work. This trait en-
compasses a range of qualities: diligence, enthusiasm, willingness,
dedication, commitment, and alacrity. In the Yoga Sutras, zeal is

called *tapas* and is one of the five disciplines (*niyamas*) of the Eight Limbs of Yoga. *Tap*, the root of the word *tapas*, refers to fire or heat. It implies a burning commitment to achieving a goal. "By *tapas*," writes renowned yogi B. K. S. Iyengar, "the yogi develops strength in body, mind, and character."[1]

Traditional *Mussar* texts refer to *zerizut* and promote enthusiastic willingness and readiness to act at the beginning of a task and unrelenting commitment and diligence toward its completion. *Zerizut* conveys a sense of what Alan Morinis calls "awakened energy," which arises when we feel inspired and dedicated to the work at hand.[2]

Cultivating enthusiasm is both deeply spiritual and critical for our *Mussar* work. Fundamentally, zeal is the enlightened directing of energy to our life's work—the greater purpose of our existence. Ultimately, the focus of our zeal is to create a better world in whatever way God or the Universe has ordained through our given talents. Pursuing fame for the sake of feeding our ego is not spiritual work or the purpose of our *Mussar* Yoga work. We do not need to (or should not) cultivate passion for work that exploits or degrades other people or resources. As long as the work we pursue has integrity of spirit, we are meant to engage in it with zeal. A gardener or a teacher who heads off to her work in the morning with passion and discipline is engaging with the Divine.

Zeal is "awakened energy."

Enthusiasm and diligence, which comprise the quality of zeal, are fundamental to transformation. Without them, the work of self-study will be limited. Every intention will be thwarted; every hurdle will turn into a dead end. Many people assume that enthusiasm and passion are organic or noncultivatable, like truffles that can only be found in the wild with the help of specially trained pigs. In fact, enthusiasm and diligence are like muscles that can be exercised to grow stronger and bigger. Enthusiasm can actually be a self-sustaining energy: Enthusiasm begets enthusiasm.

Enthusiasm is spiritual.

Your Patterns of Energy

To engage in the hard work of *Mussar* Yoga and other endeavors, we need fiery commitment and perseverance. We must be willing and available when effort is required, not just at convenient times. We need to awaken the same amount of zeal for the difficult efforts as for the enjoyable ones. And we're required to begin those efforts with passion, and then, as my college friend pointed out, maintain the enthusiasm through to their conclusion. Life sends many opportunities and obligations our way. We either respond to them with zeal or we don't.

Zeal is fundamental to transformation.

In an emergency when help is needed, do you volunteer immediately or do you wait for someone else to step forward? Some of us need to summon passion and energy at the starting point. We might be the ones who take a long time to decide whether we are willing to get involved or to help with a community project (secretly hoping someone else will take responsibility). Or we might have trouble starting new relationships, jobs, exercise regimens, or daily routines.

Some of us start out strong and passionate but halfway through a challenging task we lose momentum. We might think about quitting or we conveniently find other obligations that command our time and distract us from the original task. Many of us were allowed as kids to quit piano lessons or the soccer team when our passion ran dry. Instead of learning to stick with things and rekindle our interest, we learned to drop out.

Effort in the beginning.

Most of us who have invested a fair amount of time and energy in some activity or project get motivated when the finish line is in sight, but there are some, who, realizating that the project is 85 percent complete, pull the plug on their commitment. The last few drops of effort don't interest them and they withdraw.

To live with zeal in our lives means that we begin and sustain our energy from start to finish. Power Yoga teacher Baron Baptiste instructs yoga students to "be a yes."[3] Living with *tapas* and *zerizut* means to "be a yes." Saying "yes" doesn't just mean responding affirmatively to a task that must be done. It means offering up an energetic "yes," showing up to a task without reservations or qualifiers, and jumping in to help without being asked. Baptiste calls this quality of being "ready NOW."[4] In the context of yoga, practicing zeal means giving your best effort from the beginning to the end of each pose and each class. The work off the mat is to direct a sense of awakened energy to our relationships, jobs, and community responsibilities. We need to say "yes" and be a "yes" in this moment or any moment that is required of us.

Obstacles to Living with Zeal

What keeps us from living with zeal and sustained effort? There are many ways we can lose energy. B. K. S. Iyengar identifies dwindling awareness and focus as root causes of fatigue and loss of energy.[5] When we lack focus (*drishti*), our energy scatters. Taking on too many tasks can be an intentional or unintentional drain on our energy.

Another obstacle is perfectionism. We can become too attached to the idea of perfection and the gap between our expectations of ourself and others can dampen our passion. When we endlessly delay or postpone commitments (waiting for impossibly perfect conditions), our momentum dissipates. Or when we ask others to be perfect and they inevitably disappoint, then we emotionally withdraw. Those of us who work with volunteer organizations often see new volunteers come and go. They join the organization with idealistic dreams only to discover that the nuts-and-bolts work is drudgery or that committee work is actually akin to sausage making. Once they recognize the mundane reality, they slowly disengage.

Energy in the middle of a task.

When the work gets tough and we feel uncomfortable, we can lose momentum. Attachment to comfort (sometimes perceived as laziness) will surely hold us back. Sometimes we think that life should be easier than it is, or that if the Universe or God wanted us to follow a particular path the terrain wouldn't be so daunting.

Yet nature is full of examples of difficult treks. (Think of salmon in spawning season or migrating birds.) Whatever we are meant to do will surely require some effort and sacrifice.

Staying Inspired

I wish that I could report that my college friend's comment about my energy patterns had a lasting effect on me and that I became a zealous finisher from that moment forward. But I heard his words and continued in that same pattern for many years afterward. When we work on being diligent, we work on breaking our habits through alertness and attention. When we are aware of an undesirable pattern or habit, we can pay attention to the contexts in which it is more likely to arise. Zeal is the trait behind all our great moments of transformation.

My big breakthrough finally happened for me on my yoga mat with the help of master Baptiste teacher Tami Schneider. Tami encourages students to hold poses for long counts of breath in order to learn the discipline of staying. Every week we would go through a sequence that involved holding Warrior II, then Bound Side Angle for cumulatively long counts of breath. When you hold these poses for a long time, back to back, your quadriceps begin to shake and burn intensely—a response called "shaking and baking." Every week I would get to a certain point in the process, about three-quarters of the way, and then quit and come out of the pose. (Exactly my

Effort at the end.

pattern off the mat, too!) Finally, one Saturday morning as we moved into the sequence I made a commitment to myself to stay through the entire sequence. Those last few breaths were indeed challenging, but when the instruction came to release the final pose I was a new person. I became someone who stayed, someone who could give 100 percent from start to finish.

In our work on courage, we learned about coming out of our comfort zone. With zeal, we learn to stay outside of it. When we stay in a pose that takes us to the physical edge of our flexibility, we become more flexible. Off the mat, when we stick with reading a book that pushes our intellectual edge, we get smarter. Or on Yom Kippur when we move past our hunger pangs and keep the fast, we experience a deeper spiritual connection. Staying outside our comfort zone generates heat, as with friction, or when we work our muscles for a long time and they begin to "burn."

The core concepts of *tapas* and *zerizut* tell us we must build and maintain a fire within ourselves. We must begin our endeavors with great enthusiasm and stay dedicated and attentive to the end.

Play your edge.

Our enthusiasm yields more enthusiasm and our alertness tells us when our resolve is beginning to wane and we need to redouble our efforts.

What can we accomplish when we are willing and ready to commit fully? This trait takes us into a world of possibility. In the Yoga Sutras there is a passage about focus and effort:

> There's no value in digging shallow wells in a hundred places. Decide on one place and dig deep. Even if you encounter a rock, use dynamite and keep going down. If you leave that to dig another well, all the first effort is wasted and there is no proof you won't hit rock again.[6]

This sutra tells us that the key to success is to stay focused, don't scatter energy, don't seek perfection, stay the course, and be willing to endure discomfort. Dig one well.

Mantras

"Begin and end each task with 'yes' on your lips and mind and in your heart."

"Dig one well."

"Stay."

"Start and finish strong."

High Push-up (Plank)/Low Push-up
Chaturanga Dandasana

Plank and *Chaturanga Dandasana* work the whole body. Stay for several rounds of breaths in each pose and feel the heat begin to build in the body. Add Victorious Breath—deep and elongated nostril breathing in which the back of the throat is constricted (see page 120)—and feel the heat intensify. Work to maintain enthusiasm for the two poses from beginning to end. Plank to Low Push-up is often followed by a flow to Upward Facing Dog (chapter 10) and then Downward Facing Dog (chapter 11).

1 From Downward Facing Dog, inhale and shift your hips forward so that your shoulders are directly above your wrists.

2 Keep your tailbone in a neutral position with your belly strong and engaged. You can modify Plank Pose by dropping your knees to the mat (keeping your knees well behind your hips). Keep lifting through your belly.

3 From Plank, rotate the "eye" of your elbows forward over your wrists. Then, as you exhale, bend your elbows without dropping your hips so that your entire body hovers several inches above your mat. Keep your chin off your chest! You can enter a modified Low Push-up from modified Plank Pose, keeping your knees on the ground and your belly lifted.

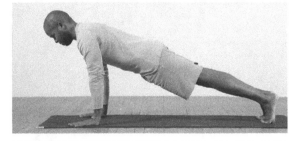

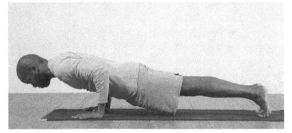

Warrior II
Virabhadrasana II

In this pose, the work with zeal comes from investing the pose with energy through the entire body and then staying and holding the pose for four, five, or more rounds of breath. Pay particular attention to the tips of your fingers. Feel them light up with energy and think of the electric-sounding Hebrew term for enthusiasm—*zerizut*.

1 From Mountain Pose, step your left foot to the back of your mat, leaving about three feet of space between your feet. The line of your front heel bisects your back heel.

2 Bend your right knee to 90 degrees, with your knee directly above your ankle and pointed over your middle toes. If your right knee is forward of the ankle, then walk your right foot further forward on the mat to take a deeper stance.

3 Extend your arms up to shoulder height, palms facedown.

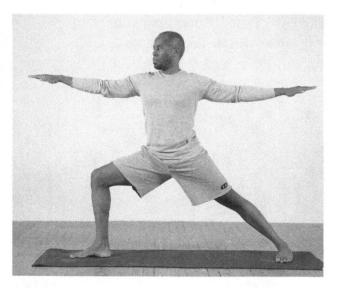

4 Level and square your hips and shoulders to the left side, while your head and gaze remain forward over your right fingertips.

5 Repeat on the left side.

Breath of Joy
Prana Sukha

A great way to increase your energy levels, Breath of Joy is a sequence of breath and movement that looks like a cheerleading maneuver or tarmac-to-cockpit communication and sounds like a Lamaze (push the baby) technique. The sequence consists of three quick inhales through the nose with arm movements followed by an exhale into a forward fold. Inhalations are known to energize the mind and body. You can practice Breath of Joy in lieu of coffee any time you need to feel more *tapas*.

1 Inhale 1: Reach your arms straight forward and up to shoulder level, and then drop them back down.

2 Inhale 2: Lift and extend your arms out to the sides of your body (shoulder height) and then drop them back down.

3 Inhale 3: Reach the arms all the way up and over your head and then exhale into a forward fold with the knees deeply bent.

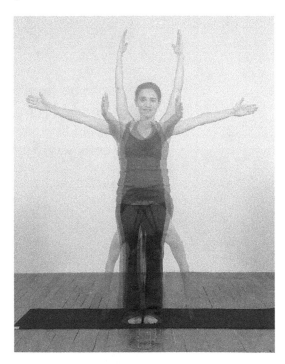

4 After the exhalation, keep your knees bent as your body rises, arms extended forward and move into Inhale 1. Repeat five to seven times. Each round takes about four to five seconds.

Explorations for Mat, Journal, and Life

1 How can you bring more disciplined heat (staying power) to your yoga practice?

2 How can you maintain a steady flow of enthusiasm from the beginning to the end of practice? From the beginning to the end of each pose?

3 What would change about your practice if you could cultivate the same amount of dedication and energy in your least favorite pose as your favorite?

4 Where in your world of work and relationships can you bring more enthusiasm and commitment?

5 How does your experience of life change when you spend a day saying "yes" more times than you say "no"?

6 How will you work on the trait of zeal this week? Does your attention need to be on starting an endeavor, maintaining enthusiasm in the middle, or finishing strong? When you bring more enthusiasm into your life, what big or small changes do you notice?

7

Simplicity

Simplicity isn't just a visual style. It's not just
minimalism or the absence of clutter. It involves
digging through the depth of the complexity. To
be truly simple, you have to go really deep.

Jony Ives

Forget your lust for the rich man's gold. All that you
need is in your soul and you can do this if you try.
All that I want for you, my son, is to be satisfied.

Lynyrd Skynyrd

A house is just a place to keep your stuff
while you go out and get more stuff.

George Carlin

Hebrew: *histapkut*

Sanskrit: *aparigraha* and *santosha*

Simplification allows us to attend to the needs of our soul. When
we long to get away, to escape from it all, to get out of the rat
race, or to go off the grid, where does that longing come from? Who

is speaking but our soul? It is asking us to shed what is unnecessary, to streamline, to pull ourselves out of the compounding complexities of daily life and connect back to the simple experience of just being … just being a soul. Our soul, buried beneath the hectic and material world, cries out to be in its true liberated state.

Recently I started leading small yoga and tent-camping retreats where participants are asked to turn off their electronic devices for the weekend and enjoy the experience of getting away from work, technology, busyness, and most other elements of what we call civilization. We eat simple healthy foods, practice yoga outside, meditate, hike in silence through the woods, read books, journal, and gather around a campfire to sing and make real-time connections with each other. The intention of the retreat is to help folks remember and rekindle an appreciation for the lightness we feel when we pare our lives down to just the basics.

Typically the pursuit of simplicity seems to spin toward complexity; finding simplicity is not simple. A trip to the local REI store clarifies this point. We decide to go camping (seeking to reconnect with nature and get back to simple pleasures) and then load up our shopping cart with equipment, gadgets, and accessories to take with us on our venture into nature. The need we all feel to get more stuff comes, in part, from what Emile Durkheim, a French sociologist in the early twentieth century, called "anomie." Anomie, he explained, is the experience of living in the modern world, which has few widely held rules or traditions. Without societal guidance, we never know when enough is enough. The yearning or felt need for more is not tempered by an appreciation of moderation; the value placed on getting more trumps the benefits of needing less. It takes diligence and discipline to work against the tendency toward complexity.

Short of becoming a recluse in a cave, how can we fight the cultural tide? We can work this trait, expressed with the Hebrew term *histapkut* (meaning "sufficient-ness" or "moderation") and the Sanskrit terms *aparigraha* (nonhoarding) and *santosha* (contentment), by focusing on six lifestyle domains vulnerable to the forces of complexity: the material world, the temporal world (time management), the technological world, interpersonal relationships, relationships with nature, and relationships with food. Overall, cultivating a sense of moderation, nongrasping, and contentment smoothes the path toward simplicity. We can feel profound change when we apply the practices of moderation and contentment to our tendencies to overdo our consumption of things; overschedule our time; become more connected to electronic communication than the live, in-person type; invite game-playing into our relationships; lose connection with the simple gifts of the natural world; and overconsume processed foods.

Six Ways to Simplify Your Life

1. Manage the Material World

In chapter 4 on order, we discussed organizing what we already possess. In simplicity we examine how we acquire such excess. Yes, everywhere you cast your gaze over your overstuffed, over-cluttered, overfilled life, you see the results of too much acquisition. Your house, garage, car, rooms, drawers, wallet, bags—they are all brimming with too many things. The material world brings complexity into our lives. Each object—clothes, furniture, appliances, technology, food, toys—must be maintained, managed, or disposed of. Then our means for maintaining, managing, or disposing of these objects must also be maintained, managed, and disposed of. (Open your closet full of cleaning products if you don't know what I mean.)

The best way to contain the complexity of the material world is by not letting it into our lives in the first place. We need to leave most of the stuff where it came from—in the store. One important path to figuring out what comes home with us and what doesn't is through increasing our discernment between our needs and our wants. *Aparigraha*, nonhoarding, teaches us to take only what we need. What do we truly need? In our lives we should meet all claims of need with a skeptical eye. When I first started practicing yoga, I hesitated to use a yoga mat. I figured that ancient yogis did not purchase Mandukas (the Lexus of yoga mats). After a few weeks going mat-less, I realized that some type of mat was essential. Over time, I've discerned that buying a quality mat is a good investment. Try practicing "going without" before you give in and buy. Another great way to practice simplicity is to ask yourself as you shop, "Is this a need or a want?" Just by asking the question, you will simplify your life.

Cultivate more contentment with what you have and you will find yourself needing less. The Jewish sages asked and answered, "Who is happy?" "He who is content with his lot" (*Pirke Avot* 4:1). Yoga teaches the same through the concept of *santosha*. *Santosha* asks us to accept everything about this moment, with its many imperfections, as enough. *Santosha* asks us to see the glass half full.

2. Clear Your Calendar

It's a fact: You can only be in one place at a time. When you say "yes" to one commitment you are automatically saying "no" to another. I know people who sit on sixteen different community and professional boards, but believe me, they are not superhuman. These busy people are saying "no" to *something* in their lives—sleep, healthy eating, exercise, family connection, or alone time. We are all subject to the same natural laws and restrictions of a twenty-four-hour day. It may be flattering or exciting to find yourself in such demand, but you should keep time available every day to pay attention to your emotional relationships, physical health, and mental well-being.

Give yourself a twenty-four-hour rule for saying "yes" to long-term commitments. Keep the word *no* by your home or office phone and computer to remind yourself to resist recruitment to additional responsibilities and commitments. Keep the Hebrew word *histapkut*, the sense of "enoughness," in mind when you consider taking on new roles. Once a year, review your commitments and prioritize them. Make sure you are spending time on the priorities in your life. Insist on getting enough sleep every night. (The Mayo

Clinic advises seven to eight hours per night for adults.[1]) Consider your exercise regimen, ideally practiced two or three times weekly, the same as the requirement to bathe and eat. Give yourself some weekly alone time to think and reflect. Remember that multitasking is a form of complication. If you're feeling overwhelmed, take the advice of a colleague of mine: "Breathe and simplify."

3. Tune Out and Turn Off

The constant deluge of e-mails, texts, calls, tweets, and updates can flood your soul right out of your life. A spiritual life, then, requires some regular time off the grid. If you just do it in irregular spurts of time, you don't let the mind completely disconnect from the busyness. Instead, designate a consistent and generous amount of time to turn off the phone, television, social media, Internet, and television at least once a week. In fact, why not unplug yourself from sundown Friday to sundown Saturday? Even if you are not a traditional Jew, or Jewish at all, unplugging for a full twenty-four hours is a very healthy practice, and unplugging on Friday is the perfect way to end the workweek.[2] My friends who observe Shabbat, by varying degrees, all refer to it in magical terms. Abraham Joshua Heschel described the Sabbath as a cathedral of time, a great and holy space—a place of serenity, safety, and otherworldliness. Shabbat is indeed otherworldly. It take us out of the world of work, errands, and busyness. When my children were small, we went to visit some friends who committed to observing Shabbat as a stay-at-home, family day. I remember very well how, as we entered their house on Saturday afternoon, we could feel a sense of profound peacefulness.

At the end of most yoga classes, students come into Corpse Pose (*Savasana*), where they are meant to lie on their mat in total, relaxed stillness. Think of these several minutes of nondoing as a reminder of both the grace and the challenge of stepping off the hamster wheel of daily life. You can create more sacred space in your practice by silencing your cell phone or, even better, leaving it with your coat and shoes.

Off the mat, use your unplugged time to connect with family and friends or spend time with yourself. Read a book, meditate, or just sit in a comfortable chair looking out the window and watch the world go by.

4. Avoid Interpersonal Drama

Living with simplicity also means staying away from game-playing and personal conflicts as much as possible. By sticking with the *Mussar* traits of honesty and silence (in the face of gossip) you can avoid most relationship pitfalls. It also helps to be less sensitive to slights and unwilling to ascribe malice to the actions of others. If someone criticizes you, let it go. In Don Miguel Ruiz's *The Four Agreements*, the second agreement is "Don't Take Anything Personally." "Even when a situation seems so personal, even if others insult you directly, it has nothing to do with you."[3] It's about them.

The *Amidah*, the Jewish daily prayer, acknowledges how disruptive others' judgment are on the peacefulness of our soul. We pray: "My God, keep my tongue from evil, my lips from speaking lies. Help me ignore those who slander me…. Frustrate the designs of those who plot evil against me. Make nothing of their schemes." Learn to be comfortable with the reality that not everyone will love you, your ideas, or your choices. Some people just like to stir the pot or feed their own ego with negative judgment of others.

5. Go Back to Nature

Going for a walk, a weekend, or a week in the woods is another way we can refresh our appreciation for simplicity. Leave all the extra stuff you think you need behind. Find relief in the simple pleasures of nature and your physical presence in it. Scientific research has conclusively found that time spent outdoors in nature offers multiple benefits for our well-being. Being in nature decreases stress levels, brain fatigue, attention deficits, and depression.[4]

When you feel the urge to get back to nature, be mindful of the influence of our consumerist culture that tempts you to buy "back-to-nature gear." Be a minimalist.

Consider the words of Henry David Thoreau in his famous book *Walden; Or, Life in the Woods*: "I went to the woods because I wished to live deliberately, to front only the essential facts of life and see if I could not learn what it had to teach, and not, when I came to die, discover that I had not lived."[5]

6. Eat Simple Foods

Moderation expressed by *histapkut* and *aparigraha* applies to your diet, too. In order to have large quantities of food available to eat in a short amount of time, there is temptation to substitute processed food for time-consuming fresh food shopping and preparation. The first step in simplifying your diet may be to eat less or add more mindfulness to the act of eating. Slowing down to actually chew and taste the food makes meals feel more satisfying and substantial.

You can also simplify what you eat by choosing foods with few ingredients. Maybe all your meals can't be simple and homemade, but for the week you are working on simplicity aim for at least one daily meal that is void of processed foods. Perhaps on the weekend you can make a whole day of eating natural and unprocessed foods. Related to simplifying our food and our connection to nature, if weather permits while you are working on simplicity, consider creating an organic garden. Plant vegetables and fruits that grow well where you live and reduce the need for pesticides or fertilizers.

Finding Balance with Simplicity

As with all the traits, simplicity requires an artful balance. While Buddhism and other Eastern religions favor asceticism, Judaism and *Mussar* frown upon wanton denial of pleasure. Although one may fast on particular occasions, fasting and other harsh abstentions from food are not meant to be undertaken with frequency or without deep spiritual regard. The Talmud instructs that we will be called to account in the world to come for any permitted pleasure we denied ourselves (JT *Kiddushin* 4:12). We are meant to enjoy whatever benign beauty and sweetness the Universe has offered.

Moderation in all things is the key—pleasure in the material world balanced by attention to the spiritual.

The final word on simplification is that it is often only when we arrive at a crisis or a personal trauma that we learn to distinguish what's truly important—what we truly need—from the insignificant and superficial. How much better will our lives be when we can tune in to the calling of our soul before the crisis or the trauma.

Mantras

"Is this a want or a need?"

"Breathe and simplify."

"Sometimes less is more."

Revolved Lunge
Parivrtta Anjaneyasana

Yoga claims that twists help cleanse the body both energetically and physiologically by "rinsing" the organs, especially the digestive tract. Whether or not this is true, you can visualize the body being wrung out of unneeded thoughts, habits, desires, emotions, and environmental toxins. The sense of cleansing generates a feeling of lightness.

1 From Mountain Pose, step your left foot to the back of the mat, keeping the left heel high and the left hip squared forward. Rotate your left leg and knee toward the floor.

2 Bend your right knee, keeping it directly above your ankle, and keep your right thigh as parallel to the floor as possible.

3 Extend your arms over your head, framing your ears. On the next exhale, bring your hands to heart center—press your palms together and twist to the right, dropping your left elbow to the outside of your right thigh. Use your bottom elbow to leverage your chest high off your thigh (heart higher than hips). Repeat on the other side.

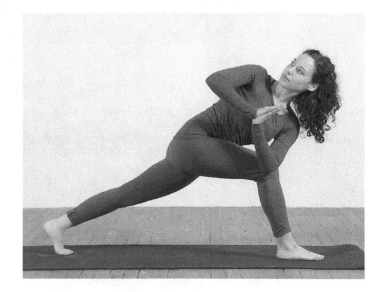

Half (King) Pigeon Pose
Eka Pada Rajakapotasana

If you spend a portion of your day sitting or standing, you're probably in need of a hip opener such as Half (King) Pigeon Pose. Hip openers help us release tension and tightness in the hips that accumulate in the typical activities of daily life. Think of the hips as storage depots of heaviness and tightness. Send lightness and breath into your hips. Let go of whatever tension you are holding on to. Explore how much you can let go of in this pose and in life. Find freedom and lightness.

1 From your hands and knees, pull your right knee to your right wrist and pull your right ankle as much as possible to your left wrist.

2 Your right knee should align with the outside of your right hip—wider, if you feel knee pain. Ideally, keep your shin parallel with the front of the mat. (Don't worry if your right heel ends up closer to your left hip.)

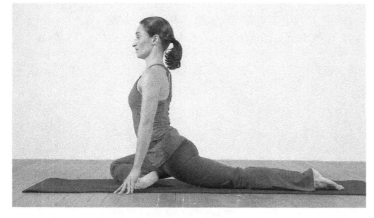

3 Square your hips forward, making sure that your left leg is fully rotated face (knee) down.

4 Hinge at your hips and fold forward, keeping your arms outstretched and hands apart. Hold this pose on both sides for eight to twelve rounds of breath.

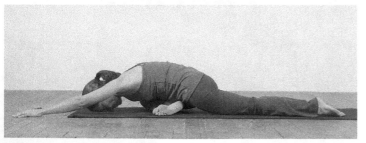

Corpse Pose
Savasana

Savasana is typically done at the end of yoga practice, when the body feels that wonderful mix of gentle energy and tension release. The pose requires total stillness, and a deep feeling of peace and surrender. It embodies the principle of "simple yet not easy."

In *Savasana* give yourself permission to do nothing. The work here is to remain in a state of not doing, just being, and finding fulfillment in that. Think of it as the Shabbat of your yoga practice. While we lie on our mat, we can find the simplicity of just breathing. We can also recognize the simplicity of our needs in this moment. What do you really need in your Corpse Pose? What do you really need at the end of the day? At the end of all your days?

1 To come into Corpse Pose, lie down, faceup, on your mat.

2 Place your feet slightly wider than hip-width apart and let your toes fall open to the mat's edges.

3 Rest your arms loosely by your sides, palms faceup—letting your fingers curl naturally.

4 Close your eyes and bring attention to any places in the body still holding residual tension, especially around the mouth and eyes.

5 Stay for a designated period of time, for the length of some relaxing music or by a gentle timer. Five to eight minutes is ideal.

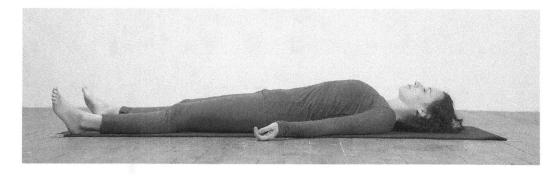

Skull Brightening Breath
Kapalabhati

Kapalabhati is a breathing technique associated with building heat and purging the body of all negativity. You can practice this breathing technique in almost any posture, but in the beginning Easy Pose, in which your spine is straight, is recommended. In *Kapalabhati*, you alternate short rapid exhalations with automatic inhalations. (In other words, focus attention on the exhalations and allow the inhalations to happen naturally.)

1 Begin with an inhale and then continue with short, forceful exhalations through your nose.

2 While making these exhalations, you can place a hand on the upper belly in order to feel the sharp contractions of the diaphragm.

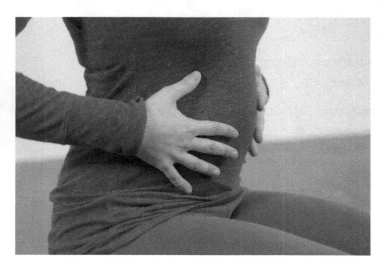

3 It is completely normal to lose the rhythm at times. When that happens, just stop and begin again.

4 Work your way into completing three sets of twenty breaths.

Explorations for Mat, Journal, and Life

1. What feels different about your practice when you keep your transitions from pose to pose simple and clean without extraneous movements? How does refraining from wiping the sweat, fixing your hair, or adjusting your clothes change the feeling of the practice?

2. How can you keep your yoga practice as free as possible from the culture of consumption? What needs can you limit or eliminate in order to practice yoga? How can you reduce clutter around your mat?

3. How can you be more mindful about what you are spending money on and purchasing throughout the day? What questions can you ask yourself when you are shopping? Are there particular behaviors, such as talking on the phone while shopping or reading catalogs, that make you more or less likely to buy things you don't need?

4. What is your relationship to your possessions and to your resources? How do they define you? How do they own you? How do they consume your time caring for them? When does caring for your possessions take precedence over self-care? In what ways do you neglect your possessions by not spending enough time taking care of them?

5. How do you glorify busyness? Are you too often selfish with your time? To whom are you most likely to be selfish?

6. What will your work on simplifying look like this week? Pick one approach to simplifying. Try to buy, be busy, buzz, or get bothered less, or get more nature or natural foods into your day. If you pick whatever seems the most challenging, you will end up choosing the simplification approach you need the most and the one from which you'll get the most benefit.

8

Equanimity

Peace. It does not mean to be in a place where there is
no noise, trouble, or hard work. It means to be in the
midst of those things and still be calm in your heart.

Anonymous

… everything can be taken from a man but one thing: the
last of the human freedoms—to choose one's attitude in
any given set of circumstances, to choose one's own way …
Even though conditions such as lack of sleep, insufficient
food and various mental stresses may suggest that the
inmates were bound to react in certain ways, in the final
analysis it becomes clear that the sort of person the prisoner
became was the result of an inner decision, and not the
result of camp influences alone. Fundamentally, therefore,
any man can, even under such circumstances, decide what
shall become of him—mentally and spiritually. He may
retain his human dignity even in a concentration camp.

Viktor E. Frankl

Hebrew: *menuhat ha'nefesh, histavut*
Sanskrit: *upeksha*

For many of us, equanimity is buried treasure. At my first encounter with *Mussar*, a short seminar, I found company in the search for more equanimity. As we moved into breakout sessions, each of us was offered one of four traits on which to focus. Three-quarters of the group chose equanimity!

I'll admit here that I have a temper that has gotten much better since I started practicing *Mussar* and yoga. Infrequently, though, it still rears its ugly, miserable head. One day, while driving my daughter to school, a car drove by my street at twice the legal speed limit. Immediately my blood began to boil and unfortunately when I caught up to the car at a very long light, I rolled down my window and "let it rip."

I could blame my reaction on reading a story in the morning paper about a woman and her two kids who had just been killed by a reckless driver or hearing on the radio that my metropolitan area has one of the highest vehicular accident rates in the country. Also noteworthy, I was already highly agitated when I got in the car because my daughter and I were running very late. I can trace my rage with the driver to a perfect storm of events, but Viktor Frankl's words—"the last of the human freedoms—to choose one's attitude in any given set of circumstances, to choose one's own way ... "—remind me that, ultimately, I am responsible for my temperament.

Histavut refers to a sameness in our reactions to both positive and negative.

I am not defined by what happens to me; rather, I am defined by my reactions to those events.

Mussar tradition directs us to equanimity with two terms: *menuhat ha'nefesh* (calmness of the soul) and *histavut* (sameness). Explanations of *histavut* generally relate back to an ancient tale regarding a student seeking entrance to an academy run by wise and mystical elders. Interviewing the student, the elders ask, "Have you achieved *histavut*?" The student asks for clarification. An elder replies, "When someone praises you, do you feel good? When someone blames you, do you feel bad?" The student pauses and then thoughtfully replies, "Yes, when someone praises me, I do feel good for a few moments, but then I let it go and when someone blames me, I do feel bad, but then I also let it go. But I never favor one or hold a grudge." The elders then congratulate the student for his good work thus far, but tell him to leave and return only when he can receive both praise and blame without any reaction at all.[1] *Histavut* conveys the quality of disengagement of the ego in the face of the words or actions of others. In light of praise or blame, a person remains calm; her soul is in a state of evenness.

The other term for equanimity, *menuhat ha'nefesh*, reflects the words of Viktor Frankl—maintaining an attitude of dignity and repose even in the most trying and desperate of circumstances. The state of *menuhat ha'nefesh* gives us the peace in which to live with more clarity and power. When our mind is unsettled, we are tossed around from one emotion to the next, depending on external conditions. One moment we hear good news and feel elated and invincible; the next moment we learn bad news and fall into the depths of despair. As we are flung from high to low and then from low to high, we lose our ability to center, to find our bearings and to make decisions from a place of stability, rather than chaos.

Menuhat ha'nefesh refers to a sense of stillness of the soul.

An unsettled soul takes us away from true inner strength and ability to connect with the Divine. *Mussar* advises that when a person's mind "is agitated, a fearful darkness falls upon him and his counsel and strength are taken from him."[2] The Babylonian Talmud has a tract that reads, "Anyone whose mind is unsettled should not pray" (BT *Eruvin* 64b). When a person's soul is in chaos, the channels of connection to the Infinite Oneness are lost.

My morning road-rage incident certainly made me feel alienated from my pure, divinely given soul. But, with the help of my *Mussar* Yoga practice, it gave me critical insight into the practice of equanimity. Equanimity means we need to be calm and to remain levelheaded and composed in the midst of chaos, not just when sitting by still waters. To find equanimity we need to be fully awake and engaged with our inner life. A state of calm creates more calm.

We practice equanimity not for the sake of achieving inner peace for ourself alone, but for the benefit of everyone. And equanimity is meant to be practiced in regard to both the ups and the downs—incredible highs and terrible lows—of our lives. The practice of *Mussar* Yoga offers tools to cultivate our inner calm.

Put Yourself in a Storm

Given a choice between a massage and a yoga class, I would always choose yoga. When I'm getting a massage, I feel very relaxed and peaceful. But as soon as the session ends I'm right back where I started. It's easy to feel calm in the sweet moments of life. The challenge of equanimity is to stay unruffled in both good times and bad.

My favorite yoga teacher offers a very physically challenging hot power yoga class, but her foremost goal goes beyond sweat and muscle. The heat and the physical intensity create a perfect storm in which her students learn to manifest an inner calm. In the middle of the class, when the physical challenge, combined with rising temperatures, are bringing our minds to a rapid boiling point, she directs our focus (*drishti*) to one narrow point, and awareness only to breath. Then, as the intensity rises further—sweat dripping and stinging our eyes, heart racing, muscles shaking, feet and hands slipping, and the room begins to feel like it's spinning—she instructs the students to watch themselves move through the wall of the storm into the calmness of the center.

> The gateway to calm is breath and a steady gaze.

One gateway through the wall of the storm is breath. Breathing and the nervous system are inextricably linked. Think about the fight-or-flight response. Perceptions of threat and subsequent fear that arise when we are stressed by an approaching bear or when dealing with a grueling work schedule accelerate our respiratory rates. We start breathing faster in response to the threat. In the midst of an emotional storm, then, our natural response is to breathe faster.

Yoga's emphasis on mindful and skillful breathing instructs students to slow down their breathing. When we move from a place of unconscious reaction to conscious breathing, we can move from panic or aggression to peace and empowerment. Slow and steady *Ujjayi* breathing (see page 120) moves our mind and body from the storm into calm. By taking ourself deliberately and mindfully into the storm, we learn to deliver ourself through the wall into the eye of calmness.

Be the Inner Witness

Equanimity teaches us to respond, not react. That's an important distinction. A response comes from a calm soul, unagitated by strong emotions; a response involves some amount of awareness and a sense of responsibility. By contrast, a reaction is akin to an eruption or explosion; it is an action without mindfulness and usually follows some habitual pattern.

Oftentimes the Sanskrit word for equanimity, *upesksha*, is translated as "indifference" or "disregard." But equanimity requires just the opposite. In fact, meditation expert Jack Kornfield teaches in *Path with Heart* that "the near enemy of equanimity is indifference."[3] Equanimity demands that we become acutely interested in what is going on inside ourself. Yoga and meditation teach us to become our "inner witness."

Another gateway through the wall of the storm is through the inner witness. Our inner witness is awake and interested in what is happening inside us. The sense of being awake and interested creates a space between an event and what we do in response to that event. Without space, we react; with space, we respond.

We can get a sense of how the inner witness works in Guy Ritchie's *Sherlock Holmes* films. Ritchie plays with camera speed—slowing it down and then zooming in to mimic the attention Robert Downey Jr.'s Holmes pays to the important clues before him. The ability to slow down and take in all pertinent information gives Holmes a superhuman ability to anticipate danger, fend off ambushes, and, of course, solve mysteries. When we are exercising our inner witness, we are slowing down our mental processes, breathing deeply, and focusing. Through the inner witness we may also seem to have superhuman skills.

Stay with Equanimity

Equanimity is a state that builds on itself. The more unsettled we feel, the more reactive we become. Instability in the atmosphere creates volatile weather events, such as thunderstorms, tornados, and cyclones. Once the atmosphere whips itself into a fury, the damage and destruction only end when all the energy has been spent.

The key to mastering this trait is to try to remain in a calm state as much as possible. Each time we lose our composure, we create an aura of unsettled energy that makes us more prone to reactivity. For those of us who are particularly vulnerable to emotional turbulence, limiting exposure to violent and disturbing films, music, and television shows is helpful. Daily meditation also helps practitioners settle their inner atmosphere.

Equanimity for Ourself and Others

Equanimity is pursued for the sake of greater efficacy and peace in the world, not for ourself alone. The inner peace we create and maintain affects those around us. When we live and share from a place of calm, we create calm in others. In this regard, we can use equanimity as a profound force for peace in our communities. Mahatma Gandhi, Martin Luther King Jr., Aung San Suu Kyi, and the leaders of other nonviolent social protests recognize the power of equanimity in promoting their causes. In fact, the juxtaposition of images of calm and peaceful protesters and violently reactive officers of the state can change hearts and sociopolitical realities.

If finding peace in our heart creates greater peace in the world, like ripples fanning out across a pond, then we should engage with it fully. But if in the name of equanimity we are simply shutting out the cries of terrible suffering as a means of seeking our own internal calm, then we are not engaging with it properly. If we are witnesses to atrocity on a small or large scale, we may seek equanimity if it promises a greater likelihood of victory against the perpetrators. But if our calm only emboldens the evildoers, then we are obligated to cultivate an inner storm or righteous rage. We must balance our desire for peace (internal and external) with the truth that "all that is necessary for the triumph of evil is that good men do nothing."[4] Or, as South African social rights activist and archbishop emeritus Desmond Tutu said, "If you are neutral in situations of injustice, then you have chosen the side of the oppressor."[5] On a daily basis we must weigh the outcome of our coming into and out of equanimity, knowing that most of the time the world prospers in a state of peace.

Ups and Downs

We tend to invoke equanimity in our responses to negativity, but the state of equanimity applies to positive events as well. When we revisit the weather analogy, we see that any disturbance to our mental-emotional atmosphere creates the same type of instability. If we shoot ourself up to cloud nine when life showers us with blessings, then we will surely rocket to the bottom when those blessings no longer come our way. Equanimity means that our soul is unfazed in the wake of either triumph or defeat.

In "The Guest House," the Sufi poet Rumi reminds us that practicing equanimity calls for us to live life in a gesture of welcoming to all experience:

> *This being human is a guest house*
> *Every morning a new arrival*
> *A joy, a depression, a meanness*
> *some momentary awareness comes as an unexpected visitor.*
> *Welcome and entertain them all!*
> *Even if they're a crowd of sorrows*
> *who violently sweep your house empty of its furniture*
> *Still, treat each guest honorably.*
> *He may be clearing you out for some new delight.*
> *The dark thought, the shame, the malice.*
> *Meet them at the door laughing and invite them in.*
> *Be grateful for whatever comes.*
> *Because each has been sent as a guide beyond.*[6]

Mantras

"Calm in your heart."

"Be the eye in the hurricane."

"From periphery to core."

"Is this worth disturbing the peace of my soul?"

Chair Pose
Utkatasana

This pose is also referred to as Awkward Pose, as it can feel quite awkward to have the hips drop and the heart lift while the knees are bent and the arms are raised. As long as you crave the desire to come out of the pose, you will not feel calmness in the heart.

1 From Mountain Pose, bring your big toes together to touch and let your heels stay a smidgen apart.

2 Bend both knees and squeeze them to- gether. Sit your hips back toward your heels until you can look down and see the tops of your toes.

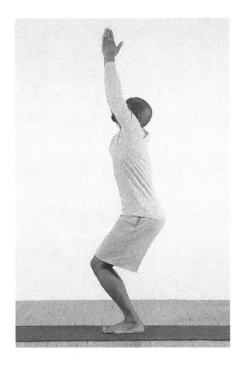

3 Keeping your shoulder blades sliding down your back, lift and extend your arms overhead, framing your ears. Broaden your collarbones and your up- per chest. Hold for five to seven breaths.

4 Use your *drishti* (focus; eye gaze straight ahead, at eye level) as a reminder to cul- tivate a calm eye in the storm.

Bound Extended Side Angle
Baddha Utthita Parsvakonasana

Moving from Warrior II into Bound Side Angle (or just Extended Side Angle) will challenge you to move through the wall of heat building in your quadriceps into a place of calm acceptance.

1 From Mountain Pose, move into Warrior II on the right side.

2 On an exhalation, drop your right forearm to your right thigh or drop your hand to your big toe side.

3 Lift your left arm straight up toward the ceiling. If you are a beginner, you can stay here or extend your arm over your left ear toward the front of your practice space.

4 Move into the bind by reaching your left hand behind your back to the top of your right thigh, for a half bind. For a full bind, tuck your right shoulder under your right thigh and reach your left hand behind your right thigh so that your right fingers grasp your left.

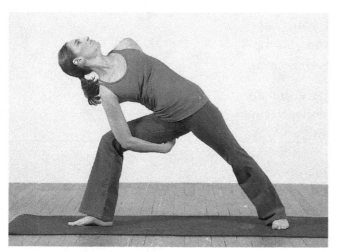

5 Stay in this pose for five to seven breaths and use steady inhalations and exhalations to find an inner peace. Repeat on the left side.

Reverse Warrior
Viparita Virabhadrasana

The challenge of Reverse Warrior is its forward and backward pull. Use the simultaneous and equalizing forward motion of your lower body and the backward motion of your upper body to conceptualize the idea of equanimity.

1 Starting from Warrior II on your right side, turn your right palm faceup.

2 Keep your torso open to the right side, while you tilt it back over your left thigh. Be mindful of the temptation to straighten your right knee; instead, bend it deeply (keeping your knee in line with your ankle).

3 Notice how the forward and backward pull take you deeper into the stretch. Stay in the pose for five to seven breaths and find peace in the middle of the tug-of-war.

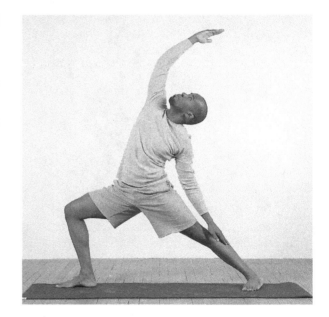

4 Repeat on the left side.

Victorious Breath
Ujjayi

Sometimes known as Ocean Breath or even Darth Vader Breath, *Ujjayi* breathing involves constricting the back of your throat while inhaling and exhaling through the nostrils.

1 To generate the constriction of your throat, practice making a big "ha" sound with an open mouth as if you were trying to fog up a mirror.

2 Then make the same breath with your mouth closed.

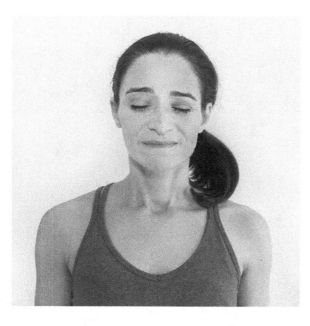

3 Engage the constriction in the back of your throat on the inhalation as well.

4 Breathe in and out through your nose and practice lengthening the breath and keeping it steady and rhythmic.

Explorations for Mat, Journal, and Life

1 As your practice intensifies, what happens to your breath? How challenging is it to keep your breath steady and even? Can you stay focused on your calm and even breath? Can you do the same toward the end of class when the intensity subsides?

2 As your practice intensifies, what happens to your thoughts? Where do they go? What feelings emerge—fear, anger, sadness? Can you identify them? Can you identify a feeling of fight or flight?

3 Notice the situations *off* the mat where you move away from equanimity. Under what conditions do you get reactive? What are your underlying emotions in those instances?

4 How will you work on equanimity this week? Can you find a way to hit the RESET button and bring your soul into a state of calmness that you can maintain all week? What are the typical daily or weekly triggers that take you out of peacefulness? Is there a particular time of day, such as in the morning when driving to work or at dinnertime, or a set of conditions, such as being hungry or tired, that challenge your state of equanimity? What mantras can you use and where can you place them in your house, in the car, or at work to help you keep your center?

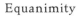

9

Generosity

At the deepest level, there is no giver,
no gift, and no recipient ...
only the universe rearranging itself.

Jon Kabat-Zinn

Is it not to share your food with the hungry and
to provide the poor wanderer with shelter—when
you see the naked, to clothe him, and not to
turn away from your own flesh and blood?

Isaiah 58:7

Hebrew: *nedivut lev*

Sanskrit or Pali: *dana, seva*

On a cold January day, my son and I were walking into Dunkin'
Donuts to buy munchkins for my daughter's birthday at
school. We were running late and when the homeless man outside
the shop asked me for "just 50 cents" I hurriedly offered to buy him
a doughnut. Instead, I got him a bagel with cream cheese and as I
stood there waiting for the bagel to be toasted I wondered why I

had placed an order that would make me even later. On the way out, I handed him the bag. From the car, my son and I watched him open it and take out the warm bagel. "Wow! Look at the smile on his face," I said to my son. "Did you see that?" My son smiled and nodded yes. Briefly, the homeless man and I made eye contact and we gave each other a thumbs-up before I drove off to deliver the doughnuts. I made it to my daughter's school ahead of schedule.

Generosity taps into the realization that we are all interconnected, bound together in our collective fates. That interconnectivity means that we are partners in the ongoing process of creating the world in which we live. When we support and care for others, we create a world in which others are caring and connected. Or we can choose to be selfish and uncaring and create a more miserable and selfish society. When we cultivate a generous heart, full of the ability to give and love, we are honoring the divinity within us.

The wise *Mussar* teachers instruct that care of others—bearing the burden of another—is nothing less than the meaning of our existence.[1] It is the feeling a parent has for a child. And the pleasure of being cared for as children motivates us to care for others as we get older. Consider how children mimic the caring of parents with dolls and pets.

Tzedakah and *nedivut lev* reflect different conditions for giving.

We take on responsibility for others, in large part, through acts of giving. Judaism distinguishes between two types of giving. Obligatory giving, which happens without positive emotional connection, is called *tzedakah*, or charity, and it is mandated by religious law. Giving that comes from the heart is called *nedivut lev*. It might be tempting to conceive of *nedivut lev* as superior to *tzedakah*, as the former stems from an internal, emotional impulse to help others. But *tzedakah* has its place, too. It frees our need to help others from the fluctuations of our transient emotions. Under Jewish law, it is mandatory to give whether you feel like it or not, because the poor are still poor even if you are not in the mood. Arguably, for nontraditional Jews, for whom adherence to all Jewish law is mostly elective, *tzedakah*, too, is essentially voluntary. When we practice generosity, we can focus on cultivating a more generous heart while also strengthening our resolve to give even when we are not moved to give.

In the world of yoga, one can make donations (*dana*) that combat the impulses of ego, vanity, or materialism. Oftentimes in the yoga world, *dana* is given in exchange for a service, such as a yoga class or a meditation sitting. Another form of generosity comes through participation in *seva*, or selfless service in which no benefit accrues to the giver. It is increasingly common that yogis are practicing *seva* by teaching in prisons, inner city schools, homeless shelters, urban ghettos in Africa, and Veteran's Administration (VA) hospitals in the United States.

More Than Money

Generosity can find many forms of expression and operate on several levels. For some folks, "checkbook" generosity—writing checks to organizations—is the totality of their willingness to share. Others give money (in the form of a bagel, discounted rent, or scholarships to college) directly to individuals in need. In our current culture, money is a vital resource, but generosity means more than just sharing financial wealth.

Seva and *dana* are both used in yoga communities to express the importance of generosity.

Most of us have lots of precious resources to offer—among them time, attention, love, wisdom, and patience. Spending time with children and the elderly who are often desperate for the attention of others can be a far greater gift than money. In India, *seva* is sometimes associated with helping with the hygiene of the poor, especially shaving, hair cutting, and washing feet. Yoga scholar Georg Feuerstein notes that *dana* includes offering blessings and spiritual teaching.[2] In that sense, prayers or the mindful sending of good wishes can be acts of generosity.

The Abundance Cycle

Mindfulness meditation teacher Jon Kabat-Zinn suggests that we approach our work on generosity with a solid sense of our own abundance.[3] We should make sure that our own needs are taken care of, that we give ourself time to relax, and that we have and appreciate healthy food and friendship, love, and a safe place to live.

An honest appraisal of all the riches in your life may surprise you. In our society we can easily focus on what we don't have—what our lives lack—especially in comparison with others. For most of us, this sense of impoverishment is a mirage that traps us in the discontent of endless wants. Practicing generosity is a way out of that trap. Generosity reminds us that we have surplus in our lives. Holocaust survivor and author Viktor Frankl recounts how even in the desperate conditions of Nazi concentration camps there were always those inmates who went through the camp offering comfort or their last piece of bread to others.[4]

> The paradox of generosity: The more we give, the more generous we become.

Once we feel and appreciate our own abundance, we can easily give to others. In turn, the more we give to others the more abundant we feel. One *Mussar* Yoga student noted that she often felt financially insecure but as soon as she began to treat her friends to an occasional lunch or dinner, she felt wealthier. That's the beauty of generosity: The more we give, the more generous we become.

As with the other traits, we need to find a healthy balance of generosity. Sometimes we can get carried away and give too much. There is a famous case of a man who lived with his wife and children in squalor after giving away his family's fortune. He also donated a kidney and desired (against medical advice) to give away his remaining healthy one, dooming him to a shortened life, dependent on dialysis.[5] Far more typically, people eventually realize that they've been volunteering too much time to a nonprofit organization or social cause and that their job or family relationships are suffering. We can also tap out our resources with one cause or organization and end up unable to support other worthwhile recipients.

Widening the Circle of Giving

As we work through this trait, we may notice that our ability to be generous has limits within particular categories of people. Some *Mussar* students report feeling more generous with family and close friends, while others find themselves more willing to give to strangers or acquaintances. Neither tendency is good or bad. They both indicate the strengths and the weaknesses of our ability to give and direct us to where our work must be done. If we find ourself shutting our hearts to the needs of strangers, we can remember the story in Genesis 18 of Abraham and other ancestors who lived in the desert and gave water, food, and shelter to messengers of God, who appeared as strangers.

On the other end of the continuum, some of us find it easier to be generous with strangers—whose faults we don't know as well—compared with people whom we know well. In the song "Easy to be Hard" from the musical *Hair*, a female character upbraids the father of their child when she asks, "Do you only care about the bleeding crowd? How about a needing friend?" and highlights the cruelty of giving precedence to the needs of real or relative strangers at the expense of our dearest family members and friends.

Letting Others Give

Many of us will gladly give the shirt off our back to someone in need, but we feel extremely uncomfortable on the receiving end of others' generosity. Perhaps our discomfort stems from low self-esteem (not feeling worthy enough to receive gifts), from how we conceive of being needy (as a sign of weakness), or because we worry about being in debt to another's kindness. Whatever our reasons for avoiding being the recipient of benevolence, we must allow others to share the benefits of practicing this virtue. There's a wonderful short scene at the beginning of *Fiddler on the Roof*, when Tevye, the dairy farmer, meets Perchik, a stranger in the town of Anatevka, and offers him a hunk of cheese for free. At first Perchik proudly

> Learn how to receive, too!

refuses to accept Tevye's gift, but when Tevye reframes his offer as a reversal of giving—that by taking Tevye's charity Perchik is giving Teyve the opportunity to practice *tzedakah*—Perchik grudgingly agrees. But like the practice of giving, we need to make sure we engage in the art of receiving with a sense of balance. Too much giving or receiving pulls us away from the ideal of moderation.

Mantras

"The more I give away, the wealthier I feel."

"The more difficult the giving, the more transformative the gift."

"Enrich others without depleting yourself."

"Accepting help is not a sign of weakness."

On the Mat

Boat with Variations
Navasana

I use this variation of Boat Pose to invoke the feeling of being of service to others.

1 Begin seated in Easy Pose, uncross your knees, and bring them to your chest.

2 Rock onto your tailbone and extend your arms to shoulder height, palms faceup.

3 Bring your feet to knee height. Use your abdominal muscles and pelvic floor muscles to keep your feet and knees lifted. (If you need extra support to keep your legs lifted and your spine

straight, you can reach your hands underneath and just below your knees, or you can place your hands on the floor behind your hip bones.)

4 From this High Boat position, exhale and extend your legs and torso as you lower your body down to hover over the mat (head, shoulders, calves, and feet don't touch the mat). This is Low Boat.

5 In Low Boat, stay for one inhalation and then on the next exhalation lift your body back to High Boat.

6 Inhale again in High Boat and then exhale and twist your torso to the right, arms extended wide (palms faceup), as if serving guests from a large tray.

7 Inhale back to center and then exhale and twist to the left (keeping your arms wide).

8 Repeat from the beginning (at least three times). Each time you extend your arms, imagine presenting an offering to someone in need. Avoid strain on your lower back by maintaining the lift and length of your spine.

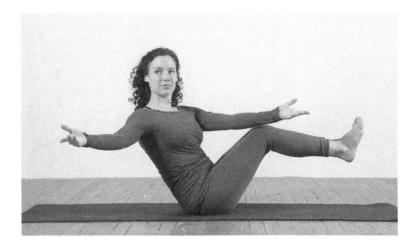

Partner Backbends

Partner work in yoga is a great way to help another yogi get deeper into a stretch. In this exercise, both yogis experience benefit at the same time (i.e., "Helping you is helping me"). While the yogi on top feels a big heart opening (expansion in the front of the chest), the yogi on the bottom gets an assist into a deeper Extended Child's Pose.

1 From hands and knees, one yogi (A) comes into Extended Child's Pose (*Balasana*) by dropping his tailbone to his heels, reaching his hands to the top of the mat, and resting his forehead on the mat. (In Child's Pose knees can be adjusted wider or narrower for greater comfort or stretch.)

2 Then the other yogi (B), facing away from A, gently sits down on A's hip bones and sacrum.

3 B lowers her spine onto A's spine. B extends her arms to a "T" position.

4 Stay in this pose for three to five rounds of breath. Partners then switch.

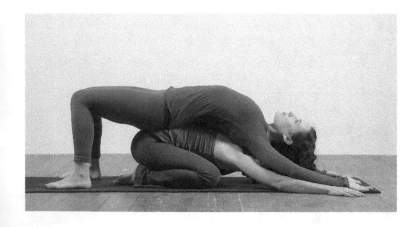

Breath Retention
Kumbhaka

What does it feel like when we block the natural process of sharing? *Kumbhaka* gives us a sense of the beauty of giving and receiving. *Kumbhaka* is not a beginner technique. If you're still relatively new to yoga, wait until you have mastered other breathing exercises, such as Victorious Breath (*Ujjayi*), Alternate Nostril Breathing (*Nadi Shodhan*), and Skull Brightening Breath (*Kapalabhati*).

Note: Never retain air to the point of strain or pain.

1 Begin *Kumbhaka* by sitting comfortably, perhaps in Easy Pose, with the spine straight.

2 Take a deep breath in and then exhale in thirds, letting a third of the air out three times before taking another deep inhalation. Do this three-part exhalation three times.

3 Then take a deep inhalation, followed by one deep exhalation. On this exhalation, empty the lungs completely and retain the air outside the body (holding the breath out). Notice the impulse that arises to begin breathing again. If you can ignore that impulse without feeling strain, continue with the retention until the second impulse arises. Release the hold by taking a deep inhalation.

4 Take two rounds of natural breath and then return to the exhalation in the thirds pattern. At the end of the third exhalation, take a deep inhalation and hold the breath in. Never holding to the point of strain, hold the breath in until the impulse to exhale catches your conscious attention.

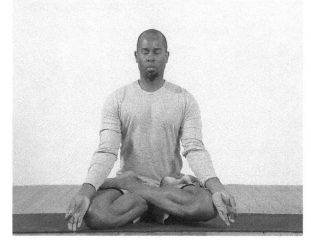

Questions for Mat, Journal, and Life

1. How often do you practice or teach yoga with a spirit of generosity? To whom are you being generous?

2. What is easiest for you to give: time, money, attention, honor, or something else? Why? What is the most challenging for you to give? Why?

3. Can you identify areas in your life in which you give too much? In what ways are you generous with yourself?

4. What is one habit of generosity you would like to cultivate?

5. How frequently and on what occasions do you allow others to be generous to you?

6. Can you identify the most specific way you can practice generosity this week? Are there particular people, or particular means (time, money, or attention, for example), that you can and should address this week? Who in your life needs more of your time? What new charity can you give to this week? Is this the week you will allow others to be generous to you?

10

Silence

Death and life lie in the hand of the tongue.

Proverbs 18:21

The silence is true and so is the talk.
Just don't be attached to either.

Rami Shapiro

What we speak becomes the house we live in.

Hafiz

Hebrew: *sh'tika*

Sanskrit: *mauna*

Silence can be delicious or ominous, depending on the context. Young mothers learn quickly that toddlers playing quietly probably means there's mischief in the making. Those same mothers, though, savor naptimes to be alone with their thoughts.

Practicing silence covers a good deal of ground and requires a fair amount of consideration. When should we be silent? When should we speak up? Is silence a refuge for renewal or a cowardly retreat? Is silence a means of giving to others, calling attention to ourself, or an unsheathed sword? What is silence—the absence of all sound or only some sounds, or the absence of noise (disturbances or fluctuations)?

Yoga Sutra 1.2 proclaims that yoga is the cessation of the fluctuations of the mind. The fluctuations are not necessarily intellectual thoughts or useful engagement of the mind with the world, such as planning, solving problems, or inventing. They are the internal chatter, the endless replay of stories and fantasies, the reiterations of the past and rehearsals of the future. A yogi's main grievance with the inner noise is that it distracts us from the present moment. These fluctuations keep us from inner stillness and clarity. Life is happening in the now, but most of us miss out on the richness of the present because we're tuned in to the chirping in our heads. Silencing the inner noise engages us more fully in life. When we practice silence, we make space to take in all that is happening in the world.

> Silence is a refuge into the present moment.

In *Mussar*, there is also a tradition of seeking silence. Rabbi Yozel Hurwitz, also known as the Alter of Novarodok, spent many years in seclusion. He spent two years locked in a room without doors, only windows for food and occasional written messages. Later he spent nine years as a forest-living recluse.[1] Rav Yozel, as he was also known, understood silence as a tool of spiritual cleansing, directing the mind to only pure thoughts.

Silence Is Golden

Silence has much value in a world filled with noise. In one sense, silence can be a retreat from the world—a way to step back and go deeper into self. On silent meditation retreats, people take vows of silence in which they refrain from talking in order to facilitate internal silence. When we quiet the external and internal chatter, we find refuge in the present. We create space to listen to ourself in the given moment. We can ask questions, such as How am I feeling now? Or what is my life purpose? In silence, there are no distractions of past or future. The quiet carves out room for spontaneity and creativity. In the clean slate of silence we can discover new ways of understanding our lives and the world. It's not coincidence that many creative people, like Apple cofounder Steve Jobs, have or had active meditation practices.

Silence can also allow deeper engagement with the world. It's not just internal chatter that distracts us from being present. Our inclination to fill up space with the sound of our own voice, music, radio, or television keeps us from hearing what is actually going on around us. When I was a kid, my family would drive out into the countryside. During these trips, my mother would insist that we turn off the radio and roll down the windows to hear and smell the natural world. Recently, I was jogging through the woods near my house when I encountered a couple walking and smoking on the path. The smoking puzzled me. Why would anyone be out in the fresh air and smoke? Then I realized that I was plugged into my iPod listening to music. Someone could easily ask why anyone would be out in the woods and miss the sounds of the birds calling, the water trickling, and the leaves rustling. You can practice the same kind of tuning in when you turn off your own talking and artificial intrusions of noise and be in the present moment at any venue: a football game, the airport, or a yoga class.

> **Silence offers deeper engagement with the world.**

Silence as engagement happens when you stop the noise and start listening to others. Turning off the radio in the car creates space to engage your children in a discussion about their day at school. When your children (or your spouse/partner/parents/friends/coworkers) are talking to you, you can be a true listener when you also turn off your internal chatter. Can you listen to what others are saying without thinking about formulating your own response? Can you keep yourself out of the conversation and just hear what others have to say? Can you hear an opinion without immediately formulating your own?

In *Everyday Holiness*, Alan Morinis directs our attention to another form of silence as it regards gossip, or *lashon hara* (evil tongue).[2] Gossip is a pernicious blight on social interactions. The reason we are drawn to it is ego, and one way we can silence our own tendencies to gossip is to address our insecurities. Not only must we not engage in gossip, but we must also create a zone of silence in the face of it. We must not give life to the gossip by actively or passively participating in the talebearing. When we are in the presence of someone who is gossiping, we can directly shut it down with a gentle reminder, we can change the subject, or we can simply walk away from the conversation. If we know that the information is false—that is, slander—we should use our voice to correct the misinformation. When confronted with the noise of gossip or slander, our moral obligation is to find some way to silence the malicious talk one way or another.

> Practicing silence is a guarding of our tongue and ears in regard to gossip.

Silence and Conflict

One of my wise *Mussar* Yoga students observed, "There is war in silence." So true. Her comment leads us to recognize the lesson of Midas: The gold of silence has limits to its worth. Sometimes in the middle of a conflict, being silent can give us space to formulate a response, rather than react with chaotic emotion. But silence can be a cold form of war. Giving someone you live or work with the "silent treatment" is just as aggressive and hurtful as hurling emotionally cruel comments his way. Silence should not be a weapon of war.

> Silence can be a form of aggression or cruelty.

Silence can also be a slow poison, as when a father "disappears" from his children's lives or two close friends don't speak for years after having a disagreement. People can cruelly withdraw from communication with people they love and care about. While silence can create a space for healing, it should be an option of last resort. Over time, silence can poison the connection and trust between friends and family.

In the face of slander, prejudice, injustice, or oppression, silence can be considered an abdication of moral responsibility. We are morally obligated to speak out and protest the unfair treatment of other people. And, to the degree that we hope and expect others to do the same for us, we must use our voice in small and large ways to upend the mistreatment of individuals and groups of people. Just recently I was involved in a conversation that became uncomfortable when one of the women began to make unfair generalizations about a minority group. Calmly and matter-of-factly I objected to the gross generalizations the woman was making. Although she remained defiant and unapologetic, I modeled for my young daughter, who was with me, the moral duty to speak up for others in the face of ignorance and unkindness. Elie Wiesel, accepting his Nobel Prize in 1986, addressed the dark side of silence: "I swore never to be silent whenever and wherever human beings endure suffering and humiliation. We must always take sides. Neutrality helps the oppressor, never the victim. Silence encourages the tormentor, never the tormented."[3]

> Silence, in the face of injustice, is an abdication of moral responsibility.

Finally, Rachel Carson, in her classic work *Silent Spring*, reminds us that silence is not the natural state of nature.[4] The world is not meant to be silent. It is meant to be filled with the sound of birds chirping, bees humming, leaves rustling, children playing, animals chattering, wind blowing, raindrops falling, and thunder clapping. Likewise, seeking permanent refuge in silence is an artificial quest. The answer to our problems is not to retreat permanently into a cave or a sensory deprivation tank without sound or distractions. Our minds were meant to fluctuate most of the time; we are meant to engage with the world. We are meant to speak with kindness and courage.

> The natural state of life is noisy.

Mantras

"Quiet the mind and be present."

"Listen to others."

"Silence gossip."

Upward Facing Dog
Urdhva Mukha Svanasana

In the pose, pay attention to the opening of the upper chest (the heart center) and the throat. Again, the heart and the throat are thought to be the energetic centers of loving-kindness and voice, respectively. The pose reminds us that heart and voice are connected; sometimes our heart commands us to speak and sometimes it compels us to be silent.

1 In a flow sequence, Upward Facing Dog follows Low Push-up (*Chaturanga Dandasana*, page 91). You can also begin the pose by lying facedown on the mat. In both cases your wrists are directly under your shoulders and your feet are top-side down.

2 As you press your hands into the mat, peel your torso off the mat and lift your pubic bone and thighs as you straighten your arms.

3 Drop your shoulder blades down your back and elongate all sides of your neck. If you like to add a small backbend, lift the sternum high before you tilt your chin upward, allowing a modest opening of the front of the throat.

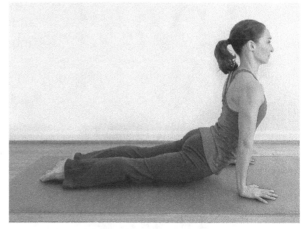

Tree Pose
Vrksasana

While holding this pose, contemplate the power of trees in their still-ness and silence. Consider the gift of serene sounds that nature often provides. Use your breath to imagine the sound of the wind moving gently through trees.

1 From Mountain Pose, root your left foot firmly into your mat and shift your weight onto your left leg.

2 Maintaining your *drishti* (focus), strong core, and *Ujjayi* breath, lift your right foot off the mat and place it on the inside of your left leg while your right knee is turned out to the right. In the beginning you can keep your right toes on the floor and your right heel above your left ankle. Over time, as your ability to balance improves, move your foot higher on the inside of your left calf or thigh (but never on your left knee).

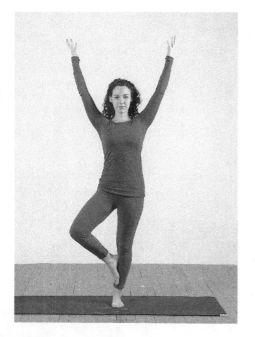

3 Bring your hands to heart center and then let your branches grow, lifting your hands directly over your head. Feel energy rise up through the standing leg and express it through the tips of your fingers. Repeat the pose on the right side.

Supine Twist
Supta Matsyendrasana

Twists are usually associated with cleansing, as they are said to wring and rinse the body physically and energetically of toxins. Considering that gossip is a social toxin, you can view this twist as a way of cleansing yourself of the desire to gossip.

1 Begin lying faceup on your mat. Your spine is long and straight.

2 Draw your right knee into your chest.

3 Extend your right arm on the floor to shoulder height, palm faceup, and then turn your gaze to over your right hand.

4 Anchor your right shoulder into the mat, while your left hand gently guides your right knee across your torso toward the left side of your mat.

5 If you cannot drop your right knee to the mat while keeping your right shoulder connected to the mat, then place a block or blanket under your right knee.

6 Hold the twist for five or more long slow breaths. Come out of the pose as you entered it and then repeat on the left side.

7 At the conclusion, hug both knees into your chest before releasing back to the mat.

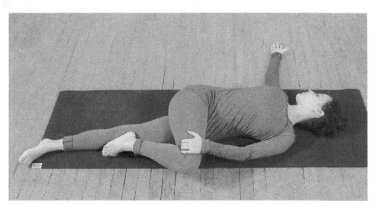

Explorations for Mat, Journaling and Life

1 How do you feel when you practice yoga in silence (without music)? And how well can you find inner silence in yoga when there is music, street noise, or other audial distractions?

2 How often do you give yourself opportunities to find safe refuge in silence? What opportunities are available to you to experience more silence?

3 How can you become a better listener?

4 Where in your life (in work, relationships, the community) are you using silence as a weapon or staying silent when the situation calls for you to speak up?

5 In what contexts are you most prone to engage in gossip?

6 How will you engage with the trait of silence this week? Will you seek more or less silence? If more silence, where can you find it—when you are in the car or going for a walk, or by silencing your own voice in order to listen more fully to others? If you'll be striving for less silence, are there opportunities this week to speak up for others or for yourself? Can you investigate whether and when you use silence as a weapon?

11

Gratitude

Enter God's gates with thanksgiving …
Psalms 100:4

Cultivate the habit of being grateful for every good thing
that comes to you, and to give thanks continuously. And
because all things have contributed to your advancement,
you should include all things in your gratitude.

Ralph Waldo Emerson

Expectations erode joy.

Anonymous

Hebrew: *hakarat hatov*

Sanskrit: *santosha*

As a child, my favorite feature of *Highlights for Children* was the
black and white "Hidden Pictures." Hidden Pictures is a game
in which you find random objects in a sketched scene, such as a
drumstick drawn among garden grasses or a spoon camouflaged

in the creases of curtains. The game suggests that among the mundane and routine, there are hidden gifts. But we must train our eyes to find them.

Gratitude in the yoga tradition is often linked with the term *santosha*, which means "contentment." But gratitude goes beyond contentment to mean something closer to appreciation and thanks. In Hebrew, gratitude is *hakarat ha'tov*, literally translated as "recognizing the good." Recently I led a *Mussar* study group, went for a walk with a friend, taught a yoga class, cleaned the kitchen, and responded to multiple phone calls and e-mails. On the surface a fairly ho-hum day, but wearing the filtering lens of gratitude I can find hidden treasures. I am grateful for the *Mussar* group because I am learning new techniques for leading discussions. The walk happened after weeks of scheduling frustrations with a friend whose company I really enjoy. For cleaning the kitchen, I have to dig deeper and I'll go with an appreciation that it didn't take too long because my husband did a thorough job the previous night. The e-mails, about projects and obligations, keep me connected to others and without the phone calls and e-mails I would feel isolated at the computer all day. In trite terms, living with gratitude means seeing the glass half full and being thankful for so much water.

But how does gratitude lead us closer to an acknowledgment of God? When I open my eyes in gratitude, I heighten my sensitivity to the kindness of strangers, a beautifully written stanza, a brilliant thought, a funny line, the poetry of nature, the calm of silence. With gratitude the world seems nicer, kinder, richer, and my life feels blessed. The cultivation of gratitude has its own alchemy. As I rediscover the bounty in my life, my soul feels a deeper connection to the Source.

Gratitude as Perspective

Yoga maven Judith Lasater tells a story that links gratitude and perspective. In a village lived a man in a two-room house with his wife, his mother-in-law, six children, a cow, and some chickens. The noise and the tumult were driving him crazy. One day he went to the village rabbi to ask for help. The rabbi listened to his tale and assured the villager he had a solution: "The answer to your problem is to buy a goat." The villager quickly bought a goat and brought it home. Now his household included his wife, his mother-in-law, six children, a cow, some chickens, and a goat. Life was even more chaotic than before. The villager again sought out the rabbi and the rabbi again assured the villager he could help. "The answer to your problem is to sell the goat," he advised. The villager immediately sold the goat and when he returned to his home the place now seemed peaceful with his wife, his mother-in-law, six children, a cow, and some chickens. The villager was grateful for the relative quiet and calm.[1]

Sometimes we need to consider just how lucky we are, no matter how difficult and trying our lives seem to be. The next time you are feeling unhappy with your circumstances, remind yourself to "sell the goat." The goat is the metaphorical burden of your chosen perspective. You can choose to focus on what is lacking or unfulfilling in your life, or you can see the abundance of what you have and be thankful.   **Sell the goat!**

Changing perspective can take on many forms, including seeing that every situation—good or bad—is temporary or an opportunity to grow.

Gratitude and Impermanence

All spiritual work involves recognition of the impermanence of everything but the Divine in our lives. The realization that everything in our midst, even the earth itself, is on loan, can make you feel a deep sense of appreciation. When my children were very young and I was trying to finish my dissertation, or maintain some semblance of a professional life, the challenge of finding a work-life balance seemed like a long shot. My grandmother would urge me to appreciate every moment because I was living the best days of my life. She would warn me that too soon my kids would grow up and move away and I would miss the mess, the noise, the neediness, and the busyness.

Now that my children are older, I realize that my grandmother was right: They were the best days, but they were also very hard. They were full of boredom, fatigue, frustration, and sadness, but also joy, laughter, love, and discovery. The truth is that all our days are the best days. These days my kids are more helpful around the house. Every day, it seems, they are more independent; the problem of getting enough time for my work has morphed into the challenge of making family time amid the competing interests of school, activities, social life, and work.

Gratitude arises more easily when you see that every situation (good and bad) has a date stamp. You may not know the exact start and finish times for your current conditions, but you can be absolutely certain that they are not eternal. So when you feel that you are going to lose your mind if you have to tell your child one more time to put his laundry in the hamper or turn off the light in her room, remember that someday those children will act more responsibly (and that will probably be the day before they move out of the house).

Everything is temporary.

Gratitude for Life's Challenges

It's far easier to feel grateful for our riches and treasures than it is to appreciate the darkness and pain of life. When I was a relatively new student to yoga, I remember struggling through classes wishing to be stronger and more flexible and to have greater stamina. What I didn't appreciate at the time is that struggle and suffering are the most fertile fields for growth.

Meditation and mindfulness giant Jack Kornfield writes: "Like the young maiden in the fairy tale 'Rumpelstiltskin' who is locked in a room full of straw, we often do not realize that the straw all around us is gold in disguise. The basic principle of spiritual life is that our problems become the very place to discover wisdom and love."[2] Tough times force us to relinquish what needs to be given up, to embrace what needs to be held closer, and to gain more insight into the nature of our problems and life itself.

I recently met with a friend who is experiencing some pain in her life—a divorce, illness, and financial burdens—and yet she was glowing. Though she was sure that she would experience dark days of uncertainty, fatigue, and physical and emotional pain, she explained that she was also absolutely certain that she would emerge from this period of her life happier, stronger, more confident, and more financially secure.

Given that we cannot avoid suffering, we can appreciate its gifts, its ability to make us stronger and more compassionate to others' suffering and to make us more appreciative of the days that are easy and full of joy. Without fear, darkness, and loneliness, we couldn't be grateful for security, light, and companionship.

Gratitude and Memory

Some people have a long memory for grievances but a very short one for appreciation. Remember to be grateful for the kindnesses paid to you and your family. Stories of immigrants to the United States who lived through the rough days of the Great Depression often include memories of one family helping another, only to be forgotten and unthanked when the recipients of that kindness become wildly successful.

Yad Vashem, the Holocaust museum in Israel, pays tribute to the "Righteous among Nations"—non-Jews who risked their lives to save Jews during the Shoah (the Hebrew word for the Holocaust), in which millions of Jews were murdered. People such as Oskar Schindler, Raoul Wallenberg, Captain Gustav Schroder (who commanded the ship of the "Voyage of the Damned"), and Irena Sendler (a social worker who help save more than 2,500 children in the Warsaw Ghetto) are honored there. While we cannot forget the unforgivable cruelty and inhumanity of so many who participated or stood by during the genocide, our souls need us to also remember and appreciate the actions of those who risked and sacrificed things big and small to help. The alternative

> Remember what others have done for you, your family, and your community.

to gratitude is bitterness and a total eclipsing of the Divine Presence in the world.

Gratitude as Domestic Currency

Sometimes we're able to appreciate the virtues of strangers more than the virtues of people closest to us. We thank the unknown person who holds the door for us when we enter our office building, but we take for granted the kindnesses of our children and partner. In *The Second Shift*, Arlie Hochschild's landmark sociological book on family, she notes the power of appreciation in the maintenance of a happy family life.[3] In the day-to-day stress of balancing work and family, and in the shadow of familiarity and expectation, it's too easy to overlook the small daily gifts we give to our loved ones and friends. Complacency is a spiritual and relationship dead zone.

Practicing gratitude feels like getting new glasses or more acute vision. We begin to take note of treasures we couldn't previously see.

Environmentalism as Gratitude

Gratitude extends beyond our relationships with people. Responding to the desperate environmental needs of the earth demonstrates our appreciation for the many gifts the earth provides. Rather than continuing to exploit natural resources, our gratitude requires that we give back in the form of caretaking. Reusing, recycling, and buying energy-efficient cars, appliances, lightbulbs—when we take these actions we express gratitude for the gifts of nature. Fossil fuels are part of the gift of nature and we need to take all gifts with gratitude and a commitment to use them wisely.

Blessings Practice

What would your life be like if you stopped taking so much for granted? How might your life change if the first thing you did when you woke up every morning was to give thanks for being alive?

In Jewish tradition you are required to say one hundred blessings a day. The routines of a traditional Jew make such a high number very attainable. Traditional Jews recite a blessing upon waking every morning, before every snack or meal, and throughout the day. There is even a blessing for when you use the bathroom, an expression of gratitude that your internal plumbing is working properly. The multitude of blessings may seem silly at first, but when you begin to take notice of the good fortune you have, you start realizing how important expressing gratitude is.

You don't need to know Hebrew or even the formal prayers to start a blessing practice. Just begin saying thanks in some form throughout the day. You can keep a tally as you go through the day or you can add them up at the end of the day. Also, if you find it hard to stop to say the blessings during the day, just run through them in your mind or note them in a journal before you go to sleep. Either way, find a way to begin and finish each day with a sense of gratitude.

Make saying thanks part of your daily experience.

Whether you begin your *Mussar* Yoga work on gratitude with a focus on gifts from the Universe, the kindness of strangers, or offerings from your closest friends and family, allow your appreciation to spill over from one setting and context to the next. Let your gratitude be boundless and abundant.

Mantras

"And this too is a blessing."

"Sell the goat."

"The best is here and now."

"Make your gratitude known."

Downward Facing Dog
Adho Mukha Svanasana

In flow yoga this pose is treated as the home *asana*. Each time we flow through the sequences we arrive back in Downward Facing Dog. The pose is in the shape of an inverted "V." In the early days of your practice, you will find Downward Facing Dog quite challenging. Express appreciation for the early days and challenges. Remember that in order to grow and get stronger you need to suffer a little or a lot. Be grateful to this pose for allowing you to grow. If you're a seasoned yogi, remember to be grateful for the respite you find in it and be grateful for the acquired strength and skill that allowed this challenging pose to become a resting pose.

1 From hands-and-knees position (shoulder- and hip-width apart), walk your hands a few inches forward.

2 Lift your hips up high and press your heels toward the floor, straightening your arms and legs.

3 Gently press your sternum toward your thighs, while keeping a slight forward motion in the armpits.

4 To make sure that you're in proper alignment, check your arms to see whether your wrists are forward of your elbows and your elbows are forward of your shoulders.

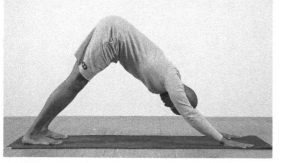

5 Then set your *drishti* (gaze) between your legs.

6 To minimize compression on your wrists, feel an energetic lift from the heels of your hands while pressing firmly into the knuckles of your thumbs and forefingers.

Child's Pose
Balasana

This is another resting pose. I make a habit of using Child's Pose as a moment to feel appreciation for my yoga practice, my relatively healthy body, the time I have to take care of myself, the skills of the teacher, the community I am practicing with, or anything else that comes to mind.

1 Come onto hands and knees with the tops of your feet flat on the mat and press your hips toward your heels.

2 Adjust the width of your knees wider or narrower for more comfort or stretch.

3 In traditional Child's Pose, your arms rest by your thighs, palms faceup. In Extended Child's Pose (pictured here), your arms extend forward, straight, and your palms typically face down.

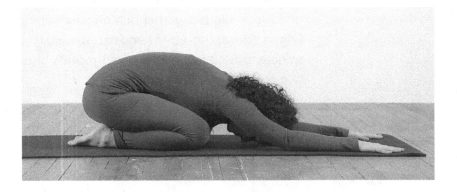

Bridge Pose
Setu Bandha Sarvangasana

In Bridge Pose, we can see that gratitude is our best connection to the past. Everything that has happened before—good and bad—has brought us to this day, this moment in time.

1 Lying on your back, bend your knees and draw your heels in as close to your buttocks as possible. (If you have knee sensitivity, scoot your heels a little farther away from your buttocks.)

2 Arms are by your sides as you begin to lift your spine off the mat, beginning with your tailbone and then traveling upward.

3 Tilt your chin slightly away from your chest to release your neck off the mat and keep your gaze on the ceiling.

4 For more intense backbending, roll slightly to your left side and tuck your right shoulder underneath your torso, then do the same on your other side. With both shoulders tucked under, bring your hands together behind your back and interlace your fingers (dropping your hands to the mat). Keep lifting your spine and hold for five to seven rounds of breath and repeat two or three times per practice.

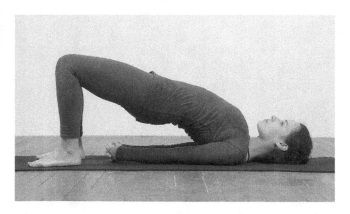

5 For a more restorative (relaxing) approach, place a block underneath your sacrum for a passive stretch of the spine.

Explorations for Mat, Journal, and Life

1 Where in your yoga practice can you feel a sense of gratitude for what is going right or well in your body? Can you identify where in your practice your body is showing up as strong, limber, and balanced?

2 How often do you feel gratitude for your yoga practice while you are practicing?

3 Off the mat, what parts of your life are working? What are you blessed with? Who is there for you in your life? In what ways?

4 The next time you find yourself in a challenging moment, how can you generate a sincere feeling of gratitude for the challenge?

5 How is cultivating gratitude a spiritual practice? To what or whom do you attribute the blessings in your life?

6 How do you plan to call attention to gratitude this week? Can you identify a specific person or two to whom you need to feel or express more gratitude? How good at expressing gratitude are you? If you have room for improvement, what steps could you take this week? Is there a particular challenge that you are experiencing in your life for which you could cultivate gratitude? Or, do you have an overappreciation for someone or something that doesn't serve or appreciate you?

12

Loving-Kindness and Compassion

Love thy neighbor as thyself.

Leviticus 19:18

Love and compassion are necessities, not luxuries.
Without them, humanity cannot survive.

Dalai Lama XIV

Hebrew: *chesed* (loving-kindness) and *rachamin* (compassion)

Sanskrit: *maitri* (loving-kindness), *bhakti* (loving-kindness),
and *karuna* (compassion)

A number of years ago I shared a true story about love and compassion with my yoga students at the local JCC. The story features a cantor, his wife, and a Ku Klux Klan leader and begins when the cantor, Michael Weisser, moved with his family to Nebraska in the 1990s. Shortly after settling into their new home, the Weissers immediately began receiving threatening phone calls from Larry Trapp, grand dragon of the White Nights of the KKK. Alarmed, the Weissers contacted the police and learned all they could about

Trapp, including that he was an invalid who lived alone. Weisser's wife, Julie, suggested that the next time Trapp called, they reach out to him with a sincere offer of help, such as a ride to get groceries. And, indeed, when Trapp menacingly called their house again, Weisser asked him if he needed some help. Trapp paused for a moment in his hateful rant, his tone lightened slightly before he declined, and then he hung up. The cantor persisted. He continued to reach out to Trapp with offers of help and a sense of compassion and loving-kindness. Then one day Trapp called the cantor asking for the type of help Weisser couldn't have imagined. Turns out Larry Trapp wanted to leave the KKK and his life of hate. The Weissers drove to his house and they spoke for hours. The story ends with Larry Trapp moving into the Weisser house as his health declined further. Julie, a nurse, took a leave of absence from work to care for Trapp in his final days. Just before his death, Larry Trapp, former grand dragon of the KKK, converted to Judaism.[1]

I still had the lump in my throat and tears in my eyes that I get every time I recount this tale when one of my students called out, "That won't work with the Palestinians." Her response initially annoyed me, but then I remembered my own resistance to the concept of unconditional love many years ago.

Oneness fills the well of loving-kindness and compassion.

While driving to a yoga class I had been listening to an NPR segment about British Nazi sympathizers. About thirty minutes later, in the middle of the class, my teacher proclaimed that "love conquers all" and directed us to open our hearts to unconditional love. My mind went immediately to the NPR story I had just heard and my heart hit a wall of resistance.

The power of love and compassion are all around us, but many of us have hardened our hearts to it. These traits are about breaking down our defenses and tapping into the potential of loving-kindness and compassion to change ourself and the world around us. What the Buddha is reputed to have said thousands of years ago—"Hatred can never cease by hatred. Hatred can only cease by nonhatred"—was reiterated by Martin Luther King Jr. when he declared, "Darkness cannot drive out darkness; only light can do that. Hate cannot drive out hate; only love can do that."[2] In a world filled with hate and war, the consequences of our capacity to extend love and care are wide-reaching.

The traditions behind both *Mussar* and yoga recognize the importance of the capacity of the heart to open. These traits are foundational qualities in both Jewish and Western yogic traditions. Kabbalists identify *chesed* and *rachamin* as two of the ten emanations of God. In the yoga texts, *maitri* and *karuna* are two of the Four Immeasurables—boundless qualities of right living.

Finding Oneness in the Midst of Differences

Loving-kindness and compassion emerge out of the highest spiritual achievement of all—the recognition of the oneness of the Universe, the divine connection among all living beings. These traits demand that we see the presence of God in the pure soul of every living creature we encounter. The root of the Sanskrit word for love, *bhakti*, means "to participate in." *Bhakti* is a love that asks us to participate in the loving relationship of the Divine to other beings. Just as the Infinite Presence loves indiscriminately, our practice of loving-kindness and compassion requires us to transcend the illusion of difference and division.

Recognizing oneness does not mean that we pretend that everyone is the same. You can't ignore the enormous lifestyle differences between you and an indigenous inhabitant of the Amazon jungle, for instance. But surely if differences among species don't affect your ability to wholly love your cat, dog, or parrot, the differences among human lifestyles, opinions, cultures, races, religions, and even values mean far less. You cannot allow relatively simple differences to obscure the basic fact that each of our souls is a piece of the Divine Oneness. Seeking the oneness, the essence of being a spiritual person, means that you set your gaze on what is shared, rather than what is not. Finding oneness opens the channels for love and compassion for all fellow beings.

Loving-kindness and compassion are companion traits, similar and often linked, but retaining different meanings and implications for practice. Loving-kindness is extended to all beings under all circumstances, while compassion is reserved for those who are suffering.

Loving-Kindness: A Two-Step Approach

From the *Mussar* tradition, we begin with the biblical command to "love your neighbor as yourself" (Leviticus 19:18). American lecturer and author Rabbi Joseph Telushkin notes that while there is nothing in the Torah that privileges the command to love your neighbor, early sages gave it primacy, as the central principle of the entire Torah.[3] Contemporary Westernized yoga, drawing on the philosophy of Eastern meditation practices, has incorporated an emphasis on *maitri* (or *metta* in the language of Pali used in Buddhist meditation) and *bhakti*. *Mussar* Yoga builds on the two traditions for developing a heart full of loving-kindness.

Love Yourself

Both traditions ask us to begin by directing our loving feelings to ourself. The biblical injunction to "love your neighbor as yourself" actually incorporates two commandments within it. First, love yourself. Second, love your neighbor. In *metta* meditations, you are always directed to cultivate thoughts of loving-kindness to yourself first before sending them to others.

The challenge of this commandment and trait is that it asks for a deep, abiding, and healthy love of self. There seems to be something about the human condition—or at least the modern Western one—that makes self-love difficult. It is a common observation that the words and feelings we express to ourself we wouldn't tolerate in any other relationship. We would never allow a friend to speak to us the way we speak to ourself. Our inner dialogue is often filled with a slew of harsh condemnations.

What does loving yourself, by contrast, sound like? Sharon Salzberg, cofounder of the Insight Meditation Center in Barre,

Massachusetts, and author of the book *Lovingkindness*, relates a story about the power of *metta* meditation. She had spent a few days at a monastery where she was called on to dedicate the entire time to sending loving thoughts to herself. She felt frustrated by the limits of the practice, yet, as she was packing to leave, she accidentally dropped a glass jar. As it shattered into tiny shards across the floor, she reflexively said to herself, "You are really a klutz, but I love you."[4]

Both traditional *Mussar* and yoga imply that the limits of our love of self limit our ability to love others. When we deny love to ourself, we cannot extend love to our neighbors. If we extend understanding and forgiveness to ourself for being imperfect and human, we will allow others to be imperfect and human. **I love me.** We all need to allow ourself to drop jars, back our cars into the neighbor's mailbox, forget our spouse's birthday, lose our car keys and cell phone, fail, fall down, get back up, fail, fall down again, and *still* hold on to a sense of unconditional love of self. Only when we can love ourself will we be able to love our neighbors when they drop a jar and back into our mailbox.

Love Your Neighbor

How do you extend loving-kindness to others? Is it merely enough to fill your heart with loving thoughts, or must you put those thoughts into action? Both *Mussar* and yoga invoke actions and emotions, but *Mussar* favors the deed over the feeling, while yoga emphasizes the feeling. Yoga addresses loving-kindness through *maitri* and *bhakti*. The philosophy of *maitri* holds that feeling and energy alone give us the capacity to infuse our words and actions with the intention of being loving and kind. If light attracts light, then the more you put out the energy of loving-kindness, the more loving-kindness will be drawn back to you, and that, in turn, will allow you to spread more warm friendliness. But the practices of *karma* and *bhakti* yoga suggest that feelings alone are not enough. The loving thoughts of Mahatma Gandhi or Mother Teresa were not enough. Their contributions to humankind came through their actions.

The *Mussar* approach to *chesed* parallels the emphasis on action, even noting that actions can precede thoughts—"to do in order to be," as the great modern sage Abraham Joshua Heschel framed it.[5] Through the act of giving, *Mussar* instructs, we transcend the illusion of separateness. We emotionally invest in those we give to, as a parent gives to and loves a child. Giving breaks down the barriers that divide us and we can then truly love our neighbor as ourself. *Chesed*, loving-kindness, is not just an emotion but also a behavior, a way of treating others with the same care and love with which we treat ourself. We must feel love and we must act lovingly. The story of Cantor Weiss and Larry Trapp demonstrates the power of acts of loving-kindness to overcome tremendous barriers and transform blind and vicious hatred into redemptive, loving connections.

Compassion:
Responding with Understanding and Action

Loving-kindness involves unconditional goodwill and concern extended to all beings. Compassion is how we specifically respond to the suffering of others. You can learn a lot about compassion by observing how you respond to your own suffering. When you are suffering, do you allow yourself to acknowledge the pain and the source of it? That is, are you kind to yourself? To practice compassion you need to learn to recognize, understand, and work to alleviate suffering. The sages of both *Mussar* and yoga teach that compassion is not just sympathy for the suffering of others but also the dedication of all of our resources—physical, mental, emotional, and spiritual—to diminish or end it.

Recognizing the suffering of others means that we are aware of their experiences. We need to be present and not lost in thought or buried in our routines. When we recognize that someone is suffering, we need to explore the nature of that suffering. We need to ask ourself—with discernment but not judgment—what is causing the person to suffer. Once we understand why someone is suffering, we can be in a position to help.

One of my strong memories from childhood centers on an evening when my father came home from work on the bus. Instead of settling down after a hard day at the law firm, he stepped inside the house for a moment to drop off his briefcase and then got into his car with a man I had never seen before. I was puzzled, but my mother explained that a sight-impaired man had gotten on the wrong bus and now my father was driving him home. When we ourself or someone else reaches out to help another person—a friend, an acquaintance, or a stranger—we see and feel the Divine Presence in our midst.

> Compassion is how we respond to the suffering of others.

Sometimes help requires inaction and here, too, we can feel the perfect unfolding of the Universe. When my daughter was young she used to raise Painted Lady butterflies. When the cocoons began to shake, she would watch the long process (several hours) of each butterfly's full emergence. The work of emerging out of the cocoon seemed arduous, and my daughter would often want to intervene on the butterfly's behalf. Over time, though, she learned that the difficult process of setting themselves free was necessary for each creature's vitality as a full-fledged butterfly. Similarly, Wendy Mogel, author of *Blessing of a B Minus*, counsels parents that they can relieve the suffering of their children by teaching them to manage failure rather than continually rescuing them.[6] Likewise, on the mat, just because you are suffering in a yoga pose does not mean that you should necessarily release out of it. If the suffering results in a deeper level of flexibility or increased strength, you should stay and just express compassion for your temporary physical discomfort.

Mantras

"Love is all you need."

"Love yourself as your neighbor."

"Widen your circle of compassion."

Pyramid

Parsvottanasana (with Head of Cow [Gomukhasana] arms)

In this challenging pose, use expansion in your chest to invoke the opening of your heart. As you fold forward, lead with your heart and surrender to a sense of unconditional love for yourself.

1 Start in Mountain Pose and extend your left leg backward on the mat about two feet away from your right leg. Right toes point to twelve o'clock and left toes are turned to eleven o'clock.

2 Square your hips forward.

3 Lift your left arm straight overhead and then drop your left hand between your shoulder blades while your right hand reaches behind your back to bind (connect) the hands (or grasp the ends of a strap or small towel to connect the hands).

4 Lift your sternum and then hinge at your hips into a forward fold. Keep your hips square.

5 Hold for three to five breaths and then take the pose on the left side.

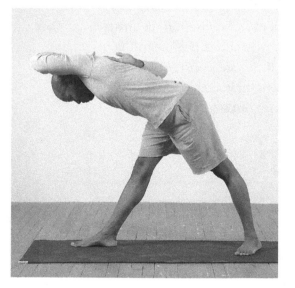
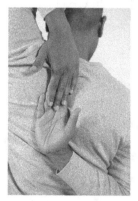

Locust Pose
Salabhasana

Another perspective on heart-opening, Locust Pose requires you to lift your heart off the floor. Let the action remind you that sometimes opening your heart to others can feel like a struggle, especially when your own heart is heavy.

1 Begin lying facedown on your mat, head turned to the right or left. To keep your legs fully rotated downward, press the tops of your big toes and your pinky toes into the mat.

2 On an inhalation, bring your head center and lift your head, shoulders, upper rib cage, arms (palms faceup), feet, knees, and lower thighs off the mat.

3 Keep your neck in line with your spine and avoid compressing the back of your neck.

4 Rotate your shoulder blades in and down your back.

5 Maintain the active energy of lifting your body off the mat and focus on the sensation of lifting and opening the heart chakra (energy center), located at the center of your chest in line with your anatomical heart.

6 Stay in the pose for three to five rounds of breath, then release your body back to the mat and turn your head to the other side (alternating left and right each time). Repeat the pose twice.

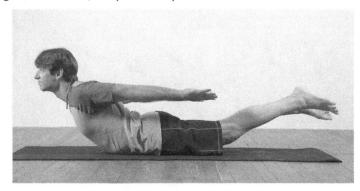

Loving-Kindness Meditation
Metta

Find a way to sit comfortably with your spine straight. Relax the typical places where you hold in tension: hands, shoulders, jaw, mouth, forehead, or some other area in your body. Begin by thinking about a time in your life when you did something kind for someone. Hold the image of yourself engaged in that act of kindness in your mind's eye and, if it feels right and natural, allow a smile or softness to appear on your face.

Still holding that image of your kind self, repeat the following silently and slowly to yourself:

May I be safe.

May I be well.

May I be filled with loving-kindness.

May I be free from unnecessary suffering.

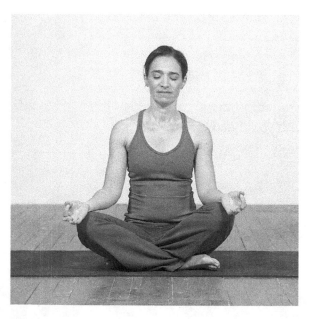

Now bring to mind someone whom you love dearly. (Pick the first person who comes to mind.) Holding an image of this person in your mind, repeat the following silently and slowly:

May you be safe.

May you be well.

May you be filled with loving-kindness.

May you be free from unnecessary suffering.

Then pick someone for whom you have neutral feelings and repeat the phrases in the exact same manner. Follow that set by thinking and repeating the phrases for someone for whom you have difficult or unpleasant feelings.

Finally, extend your feelings of loving-kindness to all beings and say to yourself:

May all beings be safe.

May all beings be well.

May all beings be filled with loving-kindness.

May all beings be free from unnecessary suffering.

Explorations for Mat, Journal, and Life

1 How can you be mindful of when you are and are not practicing love for yourself? Which poses make inner-directed love more challenging?

2 In what circumstances have you noticed the connection between love of self and love of others? Which is easier—to feel loving-kindness when you are feeling critical of yourself or when you are feeling good about yourself?

3 What element of loving-kindness or compassion needs your attention this week? Do you need to give yourself a shot of loving-kindness or do you need to work on extending it to someone in your life about whom you have neutral feelings or are in conflict? Are there people in need of your compassion?

13

Trust

And whether or not it is clear to you, no doubt the
universe is unfolding as it should. Therefore be at peace
with God, whatever you conceive Him to be ...

Max Ehrmann

Surrender means wisely accommodating
ourselves to what is beyond our control.

Sylvia Boorstein

Trust in the Lord with all your heart; and
lean not on your own understanding.

Proverbs 3:5

Hebrew: *bitachon*

Sanskrit: *ishvara pranidhana*

Trust is the art of surrendering the illusion of control. We are
asked to surrender to the power of something invisible and
undetectable, something we cannot really rightly conceive of or

easily name (God, Divine Being, the Universe, *HaShem*). It is perhaps the most challenging yet beautiful of the traits—part prostration and part poetry. In our first two or three encounters with this trait, my lovely *Mussar* group stumbled through *bitachon*, first surprised that it referred to trust in God rather than a much easier to stomach trust in other people, and then surprised again that we forgot that it referred to trust in God, "but ... okay let's see what we can do here." Trust in God or the Divine does not sit well with our times. Even in modern Israel, the word *bitachon* has shifted to mean "security" or "protection," provided not by God but by fellow humans and their secular social institutions.

My yoga teaching style favors hot power yoga, which tends to attract type A "power" people. My yoga students like to be in control. They come into class wanting the room to be warm but not too warm; they want the class to be challenging, but not too challenging; and they want music as long as it's not too "new-agey," with English lyrics, or played too loudly.

I have sat around large, small, and virtual tables with very smart, powerful, and inspiring Jewish leaders. There, too, the desire for control and the inability to surrender are very much on display. From dealing with the mundane—as with the yoga students, the temperature of the room or the coffee being served—to the more meaningful—societal shifts that make organizational life different than it was in the previous century—they struggle with the limits of their agency.

Ask yourself, How much power do I really have?

Surrender is not much in fashion in our culture. It's a tough enough sell in our current marketplace of ideas, but it's even harder to find customers in our secular world for the idea of surrendering to a deity.

You will resist this trait. You might find yourself rejecting it for several cycles or several years. But it's just a matter of time, because trust in the Divine is not asking you to do anything other than accept reality—to be in truth and at peace with the mortal limits of your own power.

Limits on Human Control

In pursuing trust we face a very big obstacle: We earnestly believe we have control—a lot of it. In our contemporary, technological world, that's an easy mistake to make. We push a few buttons and have access to information, entertainment, goods, and services that were unimaginable a generation or two ago.

Perhaps some part of the rage we see on display in Internet commentary comes from our belief that we can change other people by convincing them of the error of their worldviews. When the reality that we cannot change other people's political opinions with our well-reasoned, informed, logical, and seemingly obvious conclusions hits us fully, the contrast between the technological power at our command and our control over other people throws us into a fury. "How can I have so much and so little power!?"

If you want to change the world, said Mahatma Gandhi, change yourself. The Chafetz Chaim, one of the great Jewish leaders of the twentieth century, expressed a similar sentiment when he wrote the following:

> I set out to change the world but failed. So I decided to scale back my efforts and only try to influence the Jewish community of Poland, but I failed there, too. So I targeted the community in my hometown of Radin, but achieved no greater success. Finally, I decided to change myself and that's how I had such an impact on the Jewish world.[1]

Yet even when you change yourself, the outcome remains outside your scope of influence. You can believe that if you go to the right schools, get the right job, live in the right neighborhood, raise your children the right way, and eat the right foods, your life will generally work out well. You do have some control, to a degree. You can choose to eat healthier foods, exercise regularly, and drive without distractions because you believe that you will live a better and longer life that way. But when you look more closely at your belief, you realize that there are people who smoke and drink excessively and sit on the sofa all day long who live to a ripe old age. And there are people who did all the "right" things and died young.

How to Surrender

How can you be more open to the message of surrender? You can recognize the hurdles that get in the way of your being able to trust. Perhaps you have trouble with the word *God*. You might feel disappointed with God. You might believe that surrendering is for suckers. You may not recognize that surrendering will make you happier.

Change Names

For many people, *God* is a loaded word. It may feel corrupted by the media or by your Sunday school experiences. When I was an undergraduate, I was frequently verbally assaulted by proselytizing Evangelicals who cast a pall on the idea of God and religion for many years.

If you have trouble surrendering to God, try surrendering to a different word. The twelve-step programs refer to a "Higher Power." Even if you don't have an addiction, you can explore what a higher power means to you. Many yoga teachers refer to the "Universe" in the way that the American poet Max Ehrmann does in *Desiderata*, as an invisible, impartial, and natural force. The "Divine" is another choice that shows up, especially in mystical writings. Yoga students who are familiar with Sufi poets, such as Rumi and Hafiz, have heard God called the Divine One or the Infinite One. In Daniel Landinsky's translations of Hafiz, God is referred to as a "Master," "Innkeeper," "Beloved," and "Friend." One of the many names for God in the Jewish tradition is *HaShem*, literally "The Name" (of that which eludes our ability to understand and label). Kabbalah's mystical conceptions of God are *Ein Sof* (Everything) and *Ayin* (Nothingness).

> If *God* is a loaded word for you, find another one that expresses your sense of a higher power.

As you consider other nomenclature, try not to reject any of them outright. Instead, let them roll around on your tongue and in your mind for a few days, on and off your mat. If you cannot accept an anthropomorphic Divinity who looks like an old man, use your creative talents to conjure up your own understanding and then see what name fits best. Maybe "Infinite One" or "*HaShem*" align with your sense of the mysterious and infinite power.

The Limited Vantage Point

A classic spiritual story about trust begins with a villager whose strongest stallion runs away. The neighbors come around shaking their heads and saying, "Bad luck." The villager replies, "Bad luck, good luck, who knows?" The next week his stallion returns, leading a herd of wild horses, which the villager and his son capture. The neighbors gather 'round, saying, "What good luck." "Good luck, bad luck, who knows?" the villager responds. The following week the son is thrown from one of the new horses he is trying to tame and his leg is broken. Once again the neighbors gather 'round exclaiming, "What bad luck." And again the villager counters, "Bad luck, good luck, who knows?" Sure enough, the very next day the army comes through the village looking for all able-bodied young men, and the son's broken leg keeps him from being conscripted. Of course, the neighbors see this as a sign of very good luck.

This story reminds us that we have a limited perspective. Proverbs 3:5 tells us to "trust in the Lord with all your heart; and lean not on your own understanding." We cannot easily know what will ultimately be for the good or the bad. Our human vision is chronically shortsighted. The biblical Joseph's story of betrayal by his brothers begins in Genesis 27 as cruel tragedy. His father, Jacob, is devastated by the loss of his "favorite" son. Even if he had known the truth—that Joseph was not dead but was sold into slavery—Jacob could not have imagined finding Joseph again, let alone how the brothers' treachery would end up saving them from starvation. And, indeed, consider how the family's arrival in Egypt leads first to success (good luck), then to slavery (bad luck), and then again to emancipation and the creation of a nation (very good luck).

Who knows? No, really, WHO knows?

Surrendering means recognizing that our understanding of good and bad is eclipsed by the bigger picture that spans generations and centuries or millennia.

Surrender Is Not Passivity

Trusting in God is not an abdication of personal responsibility. It is not a free pass to indulge in bad behavior or to excuse our failures and shortcomings. I think it's fair to say that most belief systems have some fairly strict ethical and moral guidelines. Trusting in God will not lessen our responsibility for our actions. In a moral universe, we are held accountable. Turning our problems over to a higher power does not mean that we get to blame that power for all our troubles.

There's a story my rabbi told of a pious man who very much believed in God. One day, in the village where he lived, it started to rain heavily. It rained and rained, and a big flood came. A neighbor stopped by and said, "The water is rising. Come with me, my neighbor, and I'll save you." The man replied, "No, I believe in God. I really have faith. I believe." So he sent the neighbor away. It kept raining and the man went from the first floor to the second floor of his house, but the water rose until he was on the roof. Someone rowed by and said, "Get in, my friend, I'll save you. The water is rising." "No, thank you. I believe, I have faith, I trust." So the man in the rowboat went away. It rained still more and the water got up to the man's nose, so he could just barely breathe, and a man floated by on a raft. "Climb on, my friend, I'll save you." "No, thank you. I believe, I have faith, I trust." So the man on the raft went away. It kept raining and the man drowned. He went to heaven. Soon after that he got an interview with God. So he went in, and he sat down and paid his respects, and then he said, "You know, I just don't understand. Here I was your faithful servant. I was so trusting, I prayed, and I believed. I just don't understand what happened to me." And he

> Trust is not passive; it's an active decision to realize the truth about the limits of our own power.

recounts the story of his death. "Where were you when I needed you?" God looked up, eyebrows arched, and replied, "I don't understand it, either. I sent three people to rescue you."

Surrender means you must take appropriate action. In this world, "Your obligation is to act, not to determine the outcome," says Alan Morinis.[2]

On the other hand, trust also means that you get more comfortable with nondoing. When you surrender yourself to the Divine, you are acknowledging the power of nondoing. Nondoing, writes mindfulness leader Jon Kabat-Zinn, is "simply letting things be and allowing them to unfold in their own way.… Then, knowing what is, seeing as clearly as possible, and conscious of not knowing more than we actually do, we act, make a move, take a stand, take a chance."[3]

It's a bit like finding a baby wild animal that appears to be abandoned. We are tempted to intervene—pick it up and take it home—because we feel we can save it. What's usually going on, though, is that the mother is nearby getting food or teaching the baby to be independent. Our interference reflects our inability to respect and trust nature. Conservationists and animal experts will tell you to leave the baby alone.

Spiritual teacher Marianne Williams writes in *A Return to Love*:

> When we surrender to God, we surrender to something bigger than ourselves—to a universe that knows what it's doing. When we stop trying to control events, they fall into a natural order, an order that works. We're at rest with a power much greater than our own that takes over, and it does a much better job than we could have done. We learn to trust that the power that holds galaxies together can handle the circumstances of our relatively little lives.[4]

The Lightness of Letting Go

One of my favorite quotations from modern yoga pioneer Rolf Gates's *Meditations on the Mat* is this: "Let yoga be a refuge from your need to control."[5] Why *refuge*? In *Duties of the Heart*, eleventh-century rabbi Bachya ibn Paquda observed, "The worldly advantages of trust in God include peace of mind from worldly anxieties, and rest for the soul from the disturbances of trouble caused by any want in the satisfaction of bodily appetites."[6]

Trusting means letting go of anxiety, fear, and anger. The less control we have in a given situation, the more tenaciously we attempt to control. The gap between the reality of our very limited control and our delusion of substantial control underlies the anxiety of our era. When we fall for the illusion of control, we create suffering in the form of anxiety and anger.

When I was a new mom, I lived in constant worry that everything I did vis à vis my child had enormous and lasting consequences. Everything was a slippery slope of consequences far into the future. I was convinced that if he missed a nap, he'd have a lower IQ. Surely I am not the only sleep-deprived mother who believed that every choice she made had profound and lasting consequences for her child's life.

But there's nothing like a full-scale addiction to reveal how little control we have over our lives. It can literally bring people to their knees. Yoga teacher Rolf Gates recalls how his life changed for the better after he left rehab treatment for his alcoholism while serving as an officer in the military. In place of his pretense of knowing everything, he could offer the men in his unit his genuine uncertainty. In doing so, he says, he became a better listener and a much better leader. Even better, he writes, "I realized that I had been carrying an immense load on my shoulders, having to know it all, and that without this weight, life was a great deal easier."[7]

Mantras

"No doubt the universe is unfolding as it should."

"Bad luck, good luck, who knows?"

"Let go."

Forward Fold
Uttanasana

Practice this pose over and over, investing it with feelings of surrender, of bowing down with the weight of your illusion of control, and of letting go.

1 From Mountain Pose, raise your arms above your head on an inhale.

2 Then, as you exhale, "swan dive," leading with the heart and hinging at your hips into a forward fold. As you dive forward, bring to mind the sensation of letting go of a heavy weight.

3 Next, press your hands into your shins, lift your torso, and extend your back long and straight, as you come into Halfway Lift.

4 Exhale and fold forward again.

5 On your next inhale, reverse your swan dive and return to Mountain Pose.

6 Repeat the pose three to five times. Each time, ask yourself to "let go."

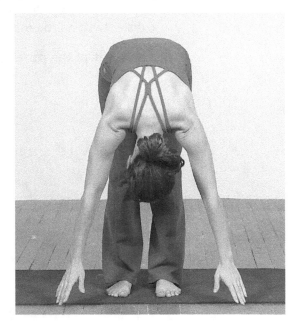

Seated Twist
Ardha Matsyendrasana

As you come into your full expression of Seated Twist, consider how, even as you twist and contort your body, the limits of your range of sight remain. You can still never see as much as you would like.

1 From Staff Pose (from Easy Pose, extend your legs straight ahead, heels on the mat and toes pointed straight up), bend your right knee and cross your right foot over your left leg.

2 You can keep your left leg extended or draw your left heel around to the outside of your right hip.

3 On your next inhale, lengthen your spine, and, turning from the waist upward, twist over your right leg to the right side.

4 Turn your neck without strain to look over the right side of your body.

5 On each inhale, think of lengthening your spine, and on each exhale, twist a little more deeply.

6 Come out of the pose as you came into it. Repeat on the left side.

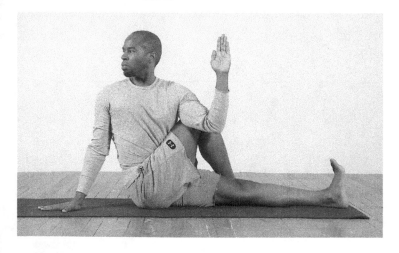

Frog Pose
Bhekasana

Frog Pose—you either appreciate it or you don't. The trick to getting the most out of it is to surrender your desire to get out of it. Recognize that letting go is not easy, and nondoing is often harder than doing. But the payoff is more lightness and ease.

Note: Frog Pose is an intense hip and groin opener and not meant for beginners.

1 Take a hands-and-knees position on the horizontal plane of the mat. In other words, face the long side of the mat so your knees can spread as wide as they can go.

2 Look over your right shoulder and make sure that your right calf is perpendicular to your right thigh. Your right ankle is directly below your right knee, and your right foot is flexed (your toes curl back to your shin).

3 Set up your left leg the same way.

4 Then press your hips behind you as far as you can.

5 Extend your spine and lower your chest toward the floor as much as you can. If you have a yoga block you can rest your head on it. This pose is not meant to be comfortable. You should feel a relatively intense stretch in your hips and groin.

6 Put a timer on and stay for an increasing amount of time every day. Begin with three minutes and increase in increments of one minute every day until you can stay in the pose for a full ten minutes.

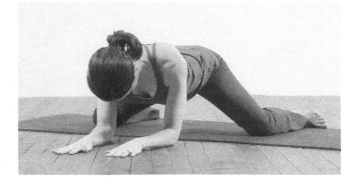

7 Come out of the pose the way you entered it.

Explorations for Mat, Journal, and Life

1 Anxiety is a marker of where in your life you are not surrendering. What anxieties are you bringing to your mat? How can you let them go?

2 How much control do you really have over the things that make you anxious?

3 Contemplate how far into the future you can really see—one minute, one hour, one day, one week? How much certainty dissipates the further you project into the future?

4 What keeps you from surrendering some of your psychic burdens to the mystery of the unknown and to the work of the Divine?

5 Although trust is a challenging trait to put into practice in one week, if you made a list of all your worries, how long would the list be? What would be on it? Can you group your worries into categories of what you can control and what you cannot? Of those you cannot control, how many can you work on to surrender to the Infinite Presence this week?

Conclusion

By your stumbling the world is perfected.

Sri Aurbindo

There is no point at which you can say that you have learned
all there is to know about your soul-traits and how they
play out in your life. There is always more to learn.

Alan Morinis

Now that we've studied all thirteen traits, we can begin to see how the development of each of them is not only important in our lives, but also fundamental for our *Mussar* practice. We need truth for the insight honesty reveals about our lives, and we need courage to face the truth and to muster the willingness to change. Humility lays the foundation for receptivity for the teachings of *Mussar* Yoga. Without order, finding the time and space for this practice cannot occur with consistency and integrity. Conversely, without the ability to let go of the old ordering of our lives in regard to how we lived out the traits, we cannot make the space for new ways of being. Nonjudgment introduces the idea that how we treat ourself and others is intricately connected, and we must live from a place that honors both ourself and others. None of our work can be accomplished without zeal—energetic, sustained commitment. Simplicity strips away the layers of unnecessary trappings that weigh down our lives and keep us from focusing on the important people and tasks in our very short lives. Equanimity keeps our souls in a place of stillness so that the light may shine steadily without flickering. When we practice generosity, we find another means of reconnecting to the real purpose of *Mussar* Yoga—to bear the burden of the other. Sometimes, we must bear that burden by staying silent and sometimes by speaking up.

Gratitude removes the conditionality of happiness and opens the door to our connection with the Divine and the wonderful gift of life. While we hold ourself accountable to transform, we must remember our duty to love ourself in the process; otherwise, we will project a harsh, critical, inner voice onto the world around us. Finally, our trust in the Divine Presence at work in the world gives us the wisdom and peace to act with due humility in the face of the limits of our power in the Universe and in the larger course of events.

After completing the first thirteen weeks of practice, you may begin to see how the traits overlap and interact. An imbalance of humility may affect our balance of courage or generosity. Similarly, an imbalance of loving-kindness may throw off our humility. Order can affect zeal; if you spend all your time looking for your wallet and keys, you will have little energy left for the big tasks, but you might need a lot of enthusiasm and discipline to put your life in order. The process of simplifying your life can increase your gratitude for what you have. Nonjudgment opens the gates of loving-kindness and compassion, and the reverse, too.

Begin Again

Perhaps you have arrived at the end of this book and feel that you are still imperfect when it comes to one or more of the traits. Indeed, perhaps you feel deficient in all the traits. I hope so! Because only when you realize and are unsatisfied by your imperfections are you prepared to keep working. The practice of self-transformation is a lifelong process. The journey never ends because you are imperfect; we are all imperfect.

This final chapter is misleading. In *Mussar* Yoga there is no real conclusion. You are meant to turn the last page over and begin your study again, and then again and again. The thirteen-week cycle repeats four times a year and then continues for cycle after cycle and year after year.

This concept of "beginning again" applies beyond the cycle of thirteen traits and thirteen weeks. Beginning again is your choice in any given moment. Just this week I was working on equanimity in the cauldron of house-guests, deadlines, and physical injury. Halfway through the week I lost my cool. In the midst of feeling ashamed and like a failure, I figured I had two options: to give in to the shame and declare defeat or pick myself up and begin again.

Both *Mussar* and yoga traditions make room for our imperfect humanness. We are meant to temper our judgment with loving-kindness and compassion. Our goal in this life is not perfection, but neither should we settle into complacency or resistance to introspection and change. When we fail—which we will, in little and large ways—we should recommit to the endeavor. We are not supposed to throw up our hands and mutter something like, "That's just the way I am." We are meant to keep practicing, to keep trying.

One critical lesson I have discovered over the years: Just when you think you have mastered a trait, the Universe will conspire to prove you wrong. As yoga instructor Baron Baptiste writes, "If you ask for inner peace, God will send you a storm in which to practice and cultivate peace."[1] Think you've mastered nonjudgment? You'll find out that your neighbor was spreading malicious gossip about your friend. Or you think you've mastered truth, and during an interview for your dream job you're asked if you've ever been fired or been issued a speeding ticket. Life is full of challenges. You will certainly be confronted by many situations that will test your growth and strength. These hurdles should be thought of as reminders that shake us out of our complacency and hubris.

Remember: You can always begin again. At any given moment during the week, you can begin again. But when you're done working on the trait for the week, it is wise to release—forgive yourself or appreciate whatever effort you've made, no matter how small. There's a saying in yoga about staying committed and keeping faith in the process: "Practice and all is coming."[2]

We will have good days and weeks, and at other times we may despair at our lack of progress. It helps to remember that, despite our continuous stumbling, our soul remains pure and the Divine Light still keeps shining within us, waiting for its brilliance to be revealed a little more every day. Why should we keep going with our practice? Because it gives meaning to our lives to radiate goodness and virtue. Because the divine soul within each of us yearns to reconnect to the Divine Oneness of the Universe—our practice takes us closer to that oneness. And when we reach for the light within us and beyond us, we give permission for others to do the same.

Creating a *Mussar* Yoga Practice Group

On occasion a new student will show up in one of my yoga classes and tell me that this is her first yoga class. As we talk, she'll let me know that she's been practicing at home with yoga DVDs for many years. I am always amazed and in awe of the student's long-term dedication—spending years alone practicing without the inspiration and support of a community.

Mussar and yoga can be done alone, but if you create a community of practitioners you'll find a powerful medium for learning. If you're practicing humility, for example, the group dynamic might raise issues of comparison or competition for you to work on right there and then. In reverse, while working on cultivating simplicity and the art of purchasing less, for example, another group member might share a thought or manner of approaching the trait work that resonates with possibility for your practice.

If you want to form your own *Mussar* Yoga practice group, all you need are a few other interested friends or acquaintances. From there you can either hire a yoga teacher to lead a yoga class or the group participants can take turns being the teacher. Group members can take turns facilitating the *Mussar* discussions or the group can designate one person as the official facilitator.

Teaching *Mussar* Yoga doesn't require you to adhere to a specific sequence of poses or a specific format. Generally, however, you would want to begin each session with a pledge of confidentiality so that everyone feels free to share personal information. The group should foster the feeling of being in a safe space. While *Mussar* Yoga is not a therapy session, it is a place where people can admit to telling a lie to a friend, being afraid to leave a relationship, or losing their cool with their coworkers. The work of the group is not to fix people or solve their problems but to help them find their own solutions by working on one or a constellation of traits.

In addition to ensuring confidentiality, every *Mussar* Yoga session should allow for discussion of the trait. The person leading the group is tasked with keeping the discussion relevant to *Mussar* Yoga. In that sense, again, it must not be run like a therapy session, where members try to address each other's problems, and no one person should be allowed to dominate the discussion. Ask questions rather than give advice. Group members can take turns leading a session that focuses on a particular trait.

Finally, every *Mussar* Yoga meeting needs to include a solid session of yoga. A short but powerful *Mussar* Yoga class can include the suggested *asanas* and breathwork for the traits, but not be limited to just those suggestions. The qualities of being humble, zealous, compassionate, or courageous, for example, can be explored in almost any pose. When we act out bravery in our yoga practice by trying an inversion or assuming a warrior stance, we know what courage feels like in the physical dimension of our being. Be sure to give participants forty-five to sixty minutes of time to get into their bodies and feel the physical sensations manifested by a trait and to understand the interplay between mind, body, and soul. Then allow the remainder of the time (at least thirty to forty-five minutes) for discussion of the trait. Allot ninety minutes to two hours total for each *Mussar* Yoga session.

As you work through the *Mussar* Yoga process, keep in mind these four "rules."

1. Fill your heart and your days with joy—let there be lightness and pleasure in the work.
2. You can begin again anytime you choose; it is never too late (but don't let yourself procrastinate, either).
3. Remember that your soul is a piece of the Divine and it is pure. You are meant to shine with the radiant light of your pure soul.
4. Working to free the light of your soul is nothing short of working to change the entire world. Be strong. Go in peace. Let your pure soul shine!

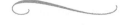

Notes

Introduction

1. B. K. S. Iyengar, *Light on Yoga* (New York: Schocken Books, 1979), 38.
2. Rabbi Moshe Hayyim Luzzatto, *The Complete Mesillat Yesharim,* trans. Avraham Shoshana (Cleveland: Ofeq Institute, 2007), 8.
3. Iyengar writes, "Yoga is not a religion by itself. It is the science of religions, the study of which will enable a sadhaka [seeker] the better to appreciate his own faith." In B. K. S. Iyengar, *Light on Yoga*, 39.
4. Originally published in his *Old Farmers' Almanac*, "The Art of Virtue" has been re-published and printed by various publishing companies, including Skyhouse Publishing (New York, 2012).
5. Immanuel Etkes, *Rabbi Salanter and the Mussar Movement* (Philadelphia and Jerusalem: The Jewish Publication Society, 1982).
6. Leonard Felson, "The *Mussar* Revival," *Reform Judaism Online* (2008); reformjudaism-mag.org.Articles/index.cfm?id=1385.
7. B. K. S. Iyengar, *Light on Life* (Emmaus, PA: Rodale, 2005), 103.
8. Baron Baptiste, *Journey into Power* (New York: Fireside, 2002), 39.
9. Alan Morinis, *Everyday Holiness* (Boston: Trumpeter, 2007), 7.
10. Ibid.
11. Meir Levin, *Novarodok: A Movement That Lived in Struggle and Its Unique Approach to the Problem of Man* (Northvale, NJ: Jason Aronson, Inc., 1996), 18.
12. Rabbi Mike Comins, *Making Prayer Real* (Woodstock, VT: Jewish Lights, 2010), 6.
13. Rabbi Akiva Tatz, *Living Inspired* (Spring Valley, NY: Targum/Feldheim, 1993), 29.

How to Practice *Mussar* Yoga

1. B. K. S. Iyengar, *Light on Life* (Emmaus, PA: Rodale, 2005), 5.
2. This concept is fundamental to Baptiste Power Yoga, created by Baron Baptiste, and elements can be found in his two yoga books, *Journey in Power* (New York: Fireside, 2002) and *40 Days to Personal Revolution* (New York: Fireside, 2004).
3. Alan Morinis, *Climbing Jacob's Ladder* (Boston: Trumpeter, 2002), 108.

1 Truth

1. Deborah Adele, *The Yamas and Niyamas* (Duluth, MN: On-Word Bound Books, LLC, 2009), 43.
2. Joseph Telushkin, *A Code of Jewish Ethics: You Shall Be Holy*, vol. I (New York: Crown Publishing, 2006).
3. Quoted by Viktor Frankl in *Man's Search for Meaning* (Boston: Beacon Press, 2006), 74.
4. Martin Buber, *Tales of the Hasidim* (New York: Schocken Books, 1947), 251.

2 Courage

1. Meir Levin, *Novarodok: A Movement That Lived in Struggle and Its Unique Approach to the Problem of Man* (Northvale, NJ: Jason Aronson Inc., 1996), 32.
2. Ibid., 33.
3. Ibid., 28.

3 Humility

1. Bhavani Maki attributes this quote to Sri K. Pattabhi Jois in his tribute to him in *Yoga Journal*'s tribute to Jois (2009), www.yogajournal.com/wisdom/2581.
2. I am indebted to Eckhart Tolle for his work on ego in *A New Earth* (New York: Penguin, 2005).
3. Marianne Williamson, *A Return to Love* (New York: HarperOne, 1992), 179.
4. Naomi Levy, Foreword, *Saying No and Letting Go*, by Rabbi Edwin Goldberg (Woodstock, VT: Jewish Lights, 2013), ix.
5. B. K. S. Iyengar, *Light on Life* (Emmaus, PA: Rodale, 2005), 36.

4 Order

1. Zygmunt Bauman, *Modernity and the Holocaust* (Ithaca, NY: Cornell University Press, 1989).
2. The equivalent Chinese term *qi* or *chi*, as in *tai chi* or *qi gong*, is more familiar to most people.

5 Nonjudgment

1. Tara Brach, *Radical Acceptance* (New York: Bantam Dell, 2003), 17.
2. Judith Lasater, *Living Your Yoga* (Berkeley, CA: Rodmell Press, 2000).
3. Lawrence A. Hoffman (lecture to Wexner Heritage Baltimore '10 Group, Chizuk Amuno Congregation, Pikesville, MD, Spring 2012).
4. Edward Feinstein, *Tough Questions Jews Ask: Teacher's Guide* (Woodstock, VT: Jewish Lights, 2012), 37.

6 Zeal

1. B. K. S. Iyengar, *Light on Yoga* (New York: Schocken Books, 1979), 38.
2. Alan Morinis, *Everyday Holiness* (Boston: Trumpeter: 2008), 125.
3. Baron Baptiste, *Being of Power* (Carlsbad, CA: Hay House, Inc., 2013), 16.
4. Ibid., 12.
5. B. K. S. Iyengar, *Light on Life* (Emmaus, PA: Rodale, 2005), 32.
6. *The Yoga Sutras of Patanjali*, trans. Sri Swami Satchidananda (Buckingham, VA: Integral Yoga Publications, 1990), 53.

7 Simplicity

1. www.mayoclinic.com/health/how-many-hours-of-sleep-are-enough/AN01487.
2. Consider joining the National Day of Unplugging every March. See http://nationaldayof-unplugging.com for more details.
3. Don Miguel Ruiz, *The Four Agreements* (San Rafael, CA: Amber-Allen Publishing, Inc., 1997), 49.
4. See this brief overview, for example: "Spending Time Outdoors Is Good for You," *Harvard Health Letter* (July 2010). www.health.harvard.edu/press_releases/spending-time-outdoors-is-good-for-you.
5. Henry David Thoreau, *Walden and Civil Disobedience* (New York: Penguin Classics, 1983), 135.

8 Equanimity

1. Rabbi David Cooper, *The Handbook of Jewish Meditation Practices* (Woodstock, VT: Jewish Lights, 2000).
2. Rabbi Mendel of Satanov, *Chesbon ha-Nefesh* (Jerusalem: Feldheim Publishers, 1995), 109–110.
3. Jack Kornfield, *A Path with Heart: A Guide through the Perils and Promises of Spiritual Life* (Random House, 2009), 190.
4. The origins of this well-known quotation are unknown.
5. Quoted by William P. Quigley in *Ending Poverty as We Know It: Guaranteeing a Right to a Job at a Living Wage* (Philadelphia: Temple University Press, 2003), 8.
6. Rumi, "The Guest House," in *The Essential Rumi*, trans. Coleman Barks (New York: HarperCollins, 2004), 109.

9 Generosity

1. Ira F. Stone, *A Responsible Life: The Spiritual Practice of Mussar* (New York: Aviv Press, 2006), 725.
2. Georg Feuerstein, *The Deeper Dimension of Yoga* (Boston: Shambhala, 2003), 370.
3. Jon Kabat-Zinn, *Wherever You Go, There You Are* (New York: Hyperion, 1984), 61.
4. Viktor Frankl, *Man's Search for Meaning* (Boston: Beacon Press, 1996), 65–66.
5. Stephanie Strom, "An Organ Donor's Generosity Raises Question of How Much Is Too Much," *New York Times* (August 17, 2003).

10 Silence

1. Meir Levin, *Novarodok: A Movement That Lived in Struggle and Its Unique Approach to the Problem of Man* (Northvale, NJ: Jason Aronson, Inc., 1996), 6.
2. Alan Morinis, *Everyday Holiness* (Boston: Trumpeter, 2007), 141.
3. Elie Wiesel, Nobel Prize Acceptance Speech (Oslo, Norway, December 10, 1986).
4. Rachel Carson, *Silent Spring* (New York: First Mariner Books, 2002).

11 Gratitude

1. Judith Lasater, *Living Your Yoga* (Berkeley, CA: Rodmell, 2000), 37.
2. Jack Kornfield, *A Path with Heart: A Guide through the Perils and Promises of Spiritual Life* (New York: Random House Publishing Group, 2009), 71.
3. Arlie Hochschild, *The Second Shift* (New York: Penguin Books, 2003).

12 Loving-Kindness and Compassion

1. www.nytimes.com/2009/01/05/nyregion/05rabbi.html?pagewanted=all&_r=0, and www.beingjewish.org/magazine/fall2003/article1.html.
2. Martin Luther King, *Strength to Love* (Philadelphia: Fortress, 1981), 53.
3. Joseph Telushkin, *A Code of Jewish Ethics*, vol. 2 (New York: Crown Publishing, 2009), 8.
4. Sharon Salzberg, *Lovingkindness: The Revolutionary Art of Happiness* (Boston: Shambhala Publications, 2011), 50.
5. Abraham Joshua Heschel, *God in Search of Man* (New York: Farrar, Straus and Giroux, 1983), 311.
6. Wendy Mogel, *Blessing of a B Minus* (New York: Scribner, 2010).

13 Trust

1. Quoted by Alan Morinis in *Everyday Holiness* (Boston: Trumpeter, 2007), 15–16.
2. Alan Morinis, *Everyday Holiness* (Boston: Trumpeter, 2007), 218.
3. Jon Kabat-Zinn, *Wherever You Go, There You Are* (Hyperion: New York, 2005, 1994), 44–45.
4. Marianne Williamson, *A Return to Love* (New York: HarperOne, 1992), 56.
5. Rolf Gates, *Meditations on the Mat* (New York: Anchor, 2002), 7.
6. Bachya ibn Paquda, *Duties of the Heart, vol.1*, trans. Yehuda ibn Tibbon and Daniel Haberman (Jerusalem: Feldheim, 1996), 361.
7. Gates, *Meditations on the Mat*, 135.

Conclusion

1. Baron Baptiste, *Journey into Power* (New York: Fireside, 2002), 37.
2. Attributed to Sri K. Pattabhi Jois.

Glossary

Asana Literally, "seat" or "taking a seat," *asana* refers to the physical yoga pose or posture. Most yoga poses use -*asana* as a suffix, such as *Tadasana* (Mountain Pose) and *Sukhasana* (Easy Pose).

Build Heat Yoga uses this term to refer to the internal warmth a yoga practitioner creates through his or her yoga practice. The heat comes from the muscular work (warm muscles) as well as some of the breathing techniques. This concept is most commonly used in flow styles of yoga that tend to keep the yoga practitioner moving from one pose to another.

Chakra A Sanskrit term that means "wheel" and refers to points of energy within the body. Yoga identifies seven chakras running from the base of the spine to the crown of the head. Each chakra is associated with a color; a lotus flower with a specific number of petals; a geometric shape; and a host of physical, emotional, and spiritual states of being.

Drishti Refers to a visual focal point. A *drishti* is a disciplined and focused gaze on one point. Locking into a *drishti* helps calm the mind, while letting the eyes move around creates more noise and disturbance in the practice.

Flow Yoga Also called *vinyasa* yoga, this is a style of yoga that links yoga poses in sequences; i.e., one yoga pose flows into another. The sun salutations are an example of flow yoga.

Heart Center In yoga, *heart center* refers to the center of the chest at heart level. The lowest point of this region is the sternum and the highest point is the sternoclavicular notch (the place where your chin rests if you drop it to your chest).

Mantra A word, sound, or group of words used to help with meditation, prayer, concentration of the mind, or religious intention. According to contemporary spiritual teacher Ram Dass, *mantra* means "mind protecting" because it directs the mind to particular thoughts. A mantra can be thought of as a *drishti* for the mind.

Midrash A Jewish form of exegesis (interpretation or commentary on biblical content) that answers questions, fills in gaps, or accounts for seeming inconsistencies in the bibical canon.

Mula Bandha Called "root" or "pelvic floor lock," *Mula Bandha* involves the contraction and lifting of the mucles of the pelvic floor upward on an exhalation. *Bandhas* are energy locks that are said to move *prana* (energy) through the body. *Mula Bandha* is also a great way to strengthen the pelvic floor to help maintain continence for both men and women as we get older.

Prana The Sanskrit term for the universal life force or energy that runs through all living beings; called *chi* or *qi* (as in tai chi or qi gong) in Chinese. The marshaling and strengthing of *prana* give us more health and strength in our lives.

Pranayama Breathing exercises in which the breath follows a specific timing, ordering, or location (nose or mouth) of inhalations and exhalations, or the retention of air in or out of the body.

Squared Hips Yoga practitioners are often instructed to "square the hips." *Squared hips* means that both front hip bones are facing the same direction, level with each other and neither side of the hip is forward of the other. Squared shoulders refers to the same alignment principle, but regarding the shoulders.

Sun Salutations There are two standard sun salutation sequences (A and B) that often begin a *vinyasa* yoga class. In Sun Salutation A, the sequence begins in Mountain Pose, and then moves to Forward Fold, Plank Pose, Low Push-up, Upward Facing Dog, Downward Facing Dog, back to Forward Fold, and then to Mountain Pose. Sun Salutation B begins in Chair Pose before moving to Forward Fold. Following Downward Facing Dog, the yogi comes into Warrior I on the right side, and then returns to Low Push-up, flowing to the next Downward Facing Dog and Warrior I on the left. This sequence also traditionally ends in Mountain Pose.

Uddiyana Bandha Called the "abdominal lock," this move involves a contraction inward and lifting of the abdominal muscles from the space just below the navel. The contraction and lift should be done on an exhalation. When done with *Mula Bandha*, it provides a strengthening of the lower abdominal muscles and is said to move *prana* upward in the body.

***Ujjayi* Breath** Also known as Victorious Breath, Ocean Breath, and Darth Vader Breath, *Ujjayi* Breath makes an audible sound. *Ujjayi* Breath typically is practiced with *vinyasa* yoga and involves inhalations and exhalations through the nose while the back of the throat is contricted, as when whispering or fogging up a mirror with an exhalation through the mouth. The friction created through the constriction is said to build heat in the body.

***Vinyasa* Yoga** See Flow Yoga.

Yetzer Hara A Hebrew term often translated as the "evil inclination." The *yetzer hara* can be thought of as impulses dictated by the ego. The sages recognize that the *yetzer hara* is problematic, but a necessary force in the world.

Yetzer Hatov A Hebrew term often translated as the "good inclination." It can be understood as our selfless or spiritual impulses.

Resources

Mussar

Bachya ibn Paquda. *Duties of the Heart*, vol. 1. Translated by Yehuda ibn Tibbon and Daniel Haberman. Jerusalem: Feldheim, 1996.

Etkes, Immanuel. *Rabbi Salanter and the Mussar Movement: Seeking the Torah of Truth*. Philadelphia: The Jewish Publication Society, 1982.

Felson, Leonard. "The *Mussar* Revival." *Reform Judaism Online*, 2008; reformjudaismmag.org. Articles/index.cfm?id=1385.

Levin, Meir. *Novarodok: A Movement That Lived in Struggle and Its Unique Approach to the Problem of Man*. Northvale, NJ: Jason Aronson Inc., 1996.

Luzzatto, Rabbi Moshe Hayyim. *The Complete Mesillat Yesharim*. Translated by Avraham Shoshana. Cleveland: Ofeq Institute, 2007.

Mendel, Rabbi Menachem. *Cheshbon ha-Nefesh*. Jerusalem: Feldheim Publishers, 1995.

Morinis, Alan. *Climbing Jacob's Ladder: One Man's Journey to Rediscover a Jewish Spiritual Tradition*. Boston: Trumpeter, 2002.

———. *Everyday Holiness: The Jewish Spiritual Path of Mussar*. Boston: Trumpeter, 2007.

Stone, Ira F. *A Responsible Life: The Spiritual Practice of Mussar*. New York: Aviv Press, 2006.

Yoga

Adele, Deborah. *The Yamas and Niyamas: Exploring Yoga's Ethical Practice*. Duluth, MN: On-Word Bound Books, LLC, 2009.

Baptiste, Baron. *40 Days to Personal Revolution*. New York: Fireside, 2004.

———. *Being of Power*. Carlsbad, CA: Hay House, 2013.

———. *Journey into Power*. New York: Fireside, 2002.

Feuerstein, Georg. *The Deeper Dimension of Yoga: Theory and Practice*. Boston: Shambhala, 2003.

Gates, Rolf. *Meditations from the Mat: Daily Reflections on the Path of Yoga*. New York: Anchor, 2002.

Iyengar, B. K. S. *Light on Yoga*. New York: Schocken Books, 1979.

———. *Light on Life*. Emmaus, PA: Rodale, 2005.

Lasater, Judith. *Living Your Yoga: Finding the Spiritual in Everyday Life*. Berkeley, CA: Rodmell Press, 2000.

The Yoga Sutras of Patanjali. Translated by Sri Swami Satchidananda. Buckingham, VA: Integral Yoga Publications, 1990.

Jewish Spirituality

Buber, Martin. *Tales of the Hasidim*. New York: Schocken Books, 1947.

———. *Way of Man: According to Hasidic Teaching*. Woodstock, VT: Jewish Lights, 2012.

Comins, Rabbi Mike. *Making Prayer Real: Leading Jewish Spiritual Voices on Why Prayer Is Difficult and What to Do about It*. Woodstock, VT: Jewish Lights, 2010.

Cooper, David A. *God Is a Verb: Kabbalah and the Practice of Mystical Judaism.* New York: Riverside Books, 1997.

————. *The Handbook of Jewish Meditation Practices: A Guide to Enriching the Sabbath and Other Days of Your Life.* Woodstock, VT: Jewish Lights, 2000.

Heschel, Abraham Joshua. *God in Search of Man: A Philosophy of Judaism.* New York: Farrar, Straus and Giroux, 1983.

————. *The Sabbath.* New York: Farrar, Straus and Giroux, 1995.

Matt, Daniel. *God and the Big Bang: Discovering Harmony Between Science and Spirituality.* Woodstock, VT: Jewish Lights, 2006.

Shapiro, Rami. *Hasidic Tales: Annotated and Explained.* Woodstock, VT: SkyLight Paths, 2011.

Tatz, Rabbi Akiva. *Living Inspired.* Southfield, MI: Targum/Feldheim, 1993.

Telushkin, Joseph. *A Code of Jewish Ethics*, vols. 1 and 2. New York: Crown Publishing, 2009.

Other Spirituality

Brach, Tara. *Radical Acceptance: Embracing Your Life with the Heart of a Buddha.* New York: Bantam Dell, 2003.

Frankl, Vicktor. *Man's Search for Meaning.* Boston: Beacon Press, 1996.

Kabat-Zinn, Jon. *Wherever You Go, There You Are: Mindfulness Meditation in Everyday Life.* New York: Hyperion, 1984.

Kornfield, Jack. *A Path with Heart: A Guide Through the Perils and Promises of Spiritual Life.* New York: Random House, 2009.

Ruiz, Don Miguel. *The Four Agreements.* San Rafael, CA: Amber-Allen Publishing, 1997.

Salzberg, Sharon. *Lovingkindness: The Revolutionary Art of Happiness.* Boston: Shambhala Publications, 2011.

Tolle, Eckhart. *A New Earth: Awakening to Your Life's Purpose.* New York: Penguin, 2005.

Williamson, Marianne. *A Return to Love: Reflections on the Principles of "A Course in Miracles."* New York: HarperOne, 1992.

Additional Resources

Bauman, Zygmunt. *Modernity and the Holocaust.* Ithaca, NY: Cornell University Press, 1989.

Carson, Rachel. *Silent Spring.* New York: First Mariner Books, 2002.

Franklin, Benjamin. *The Art of Virtue.* New York: Skyhouse Publishing, 2012.

Hafiz. *The Gift.* Translated by Daniel Landinsky. New York: Penguin, 1999.

Hochschild, Arlie. *The Second Shift: Working Families and the Revolution at Home.* New York: Penguin Books, 2003.

Issacson, Walter. *Steve Jobs.* New York: Simon & Schuster, 2011.

King, Martin Luther Jr. *Strength to Love.* Philadelphia: Fortress, 1981.

Mogel, Wendy. *Blessing of a B Minus: Using Jewish Teachings to Raise Resilient Teenagers.* New York: Scribner, 2010.

Rumi, Jalal al-Din. *The Essential Rumi.* Translated by Coleman Barks. New York: HarperCollins, 2004.

Thoreau, Henry David. *Walden and Civil Disobedience.* New York: Penguin Classics, 1983.

Notes

Notes

Notes

Notes

Bible Study / Midrash

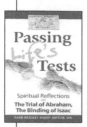

Passing Life's Tests: Spiritual Reflections on the Trial of Abraham, the Binding of Isaac   *By Rabbi Bradley Shavit Artson, DHL*
Invites us to use this powerful tale as a tool for our own soul wrestling, to confront our existential sacrifices and enable us to face—and surmount—life's tests.
6 x 9, 176 pp, Quality PB, 978-1-58023-631-7 **$18.99**

The Messiah and the Jews: Three Thousand Years of Tradition, Belief and Hope   *By Rabbi Elaine Rose Glickman; Foreword by Rabbi Neil Gillman, PhD; Preface by Rabbi Judith Z. Abrams, PhD*
Explores and explains an astonishing range of primary and secondary sources, infusing them with new meaning for the modern reader.
6 x 9, 192 pp, Quality PB, 978-1-58023-690-4 **$16.99**

Speaking Torah: Spiritual Teachings from around the Maggid's Table—in Two Volumes   *By Arthur Green, with Ebn Leader, Ariel Evan Mayse and Or N. Rose*
The most powerful Hasidic teachings made accessible—from some of the world's preeminent authorities on Jewish thought and spirituality.
Volume 1—6 x 9, 512 pp, Hardcover, 978-1-58023-668-3 **$34.99**
Volume 2—6 x 9, 448 pp, Hardcover, 978-1-58023-694-2 **$34.99**

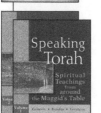

Masking and Unmasking Ourselves: Interpreting Biblical Texts on Clothing & Identity   *By Dr. Norman J. Cohen*
Presents ten Bible stories that involve clothing in an essential way, as a means of learning about the text, its characters and their interactions.
6 x 9, 240 pp, HC, 978-1-58023-461-0 **$24.99**

The Genesis of Leadership: What the Bible Teaches Us about Vision, Values and Leading Change   *By Rabbi Nathan Laufer; Foreword by Senator Joseph I. Lieberman*
6 x 9, 288 pp, Quality PB, 978-1-58023-352-1 **$18.99**

Hineini in Our Lives: Learning How to Respond to Others through 14 Biblical Texts and Personal Stories   *By Rabbi Norman J. Cohen, PhD*   6 x 9, 240 pp, Quality PB, 978-1-58023-274-6 **$16.99**

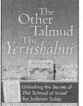

The Modern Men's Torah Commentary: New Insights from Jewish Men on the 54 Weekly Torah Portions   *Edited by Rabbi Jeffrey K. Salkin*
6 x 9, 368 pp, HC, 978-1-58023-395-8 **$24.99**

Moses and the Journey to Leadership: Timeless Lessons of Effective Management from the Bible and Today's Leaders   *By Rabbi Norman J. Cohen, PhD*
6 x 9, 240 pp, Quality PB, 978-1-58023-351-4 **$18.99**; HC, 978-1-58023-227-2 **$21.99**

The Other Talmud—The *Yerushalmi*: Unlocking the Secrets of *The Talmud of Israel* for Judaism Today   *By Rabbi Judith Z. Abrams, PhD*
6 x 9, 256 pp, HC, 978-1-58023-463-4 **$24.99**

Sage Tales: Wisdom and Wonder from the Rabbis of the Talmud
By Rabbi Burton L. Visotzky   6 x 9, 256 pp, HC, 978-1-58023-456-6 **$24.99**

The Torah Revolution: Fourteen Truths That Changed the World
By Rabbi Reuven Hammer, PhD   6 x 9, 240 pp, HC, 978-1-58023-457-3 **$24.99**

The Wisdom of Judaism: An Introduction to the Values of the Talmud
By Rabbi Dov Peretz Elkins   6 x 9, 192 pp, Quality PB, 978-1-58023-327-9 **$16.99**

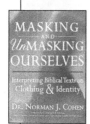

Congregation Resources

Jewish Megatrends: Charting the Course of the American Jewish Future
By Rabbi Sidney Schwarz; Foreword by Ambassador Stuart E. Eizenstat
Visionary solutions for a community ripe for transformational change—from fourteen leading innovators of Jewish life.
6 x 9, 288 pp, HC, 978-1-58023-667-6 **$24.99**

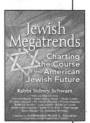

Relational Judaism: Using the Power of Relationships to Transform the Jewish Community *By Dr. Ron Wolfson*
How to transform the model of twentieth-century Jewish institutions into twenty-first-century relational communities offering meaning and purpose, belonging and blessing.
6 x 9, 288 pp, HC, 978-1-58023-666-9 **$24.99**

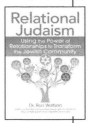

Revolution of Jewish Spirit: How to Revive *Ruakh* in Your Spiritual Life, Transform Your Synagogue & Inspire Your Jewish Community
By Rabbi Baruch HaLevi, DMin, and Ellen Frankel, LCSW; Foreword by Dr. Ron Wolfson
A practical and engaging guide to reinvigorating Jewish life. Offers strategies for sustaining and expanding transformation, impassioned leadership, inspired programming and inviting sacred spaces.
6 x 9, 224 pp, Quality PB Original, 978-1-58023-625-6 **$19.99**

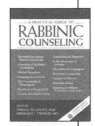

Building a Successful Volunteer Culture: Finding Meaning in Service in the Jewish Community *By Rabbi Charles Simon; Foreword by Shelley Lindauer; Preface by Dr. Ron Wolfson*
6 x 9, 192 pp, Quality PB, 978-1-58023-408-5 **$16.99**

The Case for Jewish Peoplehood: Can We Be One?
By Dr. Erica Brown and Dr. Misha Galperin; Foreword by Rabbi Joseph Telushkin
6 x 9, 224 pp, HC, 978-1-58023-401-6 **$21.99**

Empowered Judaism: What Independent Minyanim Can Teach Us about Building Vibrant Jewish Communities *By Rabbi Elie Kaunfer; Foreword by Prof. Jonathan D. Sarna*
6 x 9, 224 pp, Quality PB, 978-1-58023-412-2 **$18.99**

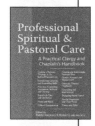

Finding a Spiritual Home: How a New Generation of Jews Can Transform the American Synagogue *By Rabbi Sidney Schwarz*
6 x 9, 352 pp, Quality PB, 978-1-58023-185-5 **$19.95**

Inspired Jewish Leadership: Practical Approaches to Building Strong Communities
By Dr. Erica Brown 6 x 9, 256 pp, HC, 978-1-58023-361-3 **$27.99**

Jewish Pastoral Care, 2nd Edition: A Practical Handbook from Traditional & Contemporary Sources *Edited by Rabbi Dayle A. Friedman, MSW, MAJCS, BCC*
6 x 9, 528 pp, Quality PB, 978-1-58023-427-6 **$35.00**

Jewish Spiritual Direction: An Innovative Guide from Traditional and Contemporary Sources
Edited by Rabbi Howard A. Addison, PhD, and Barbara Eve Breitman, MSW
6 x 9, 368 pp, HC, 978-1-58023-230-2 **$30.00**

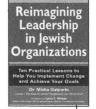

A Practical Guide to Rabbinic Counseling
Edited by Rabbi Yisrael N. Levitz, PhD, and Rabbi Abraham J. Twerski, MD
6 x 9, 432 pp, HC, 978-1-58023-562-4 **$40.00**

Professional Spiritual & Pastoral Care: A Practical Clergy and Chaplain's Handbook
Edited by Rabbi Stephen B. Roberts, MBA, MHL, BCJC
6 x 9, 480 pp, HC, 978-1-59473-312-3 **$50.00**

Reimagining Leadership in Jewish Organizations: Ten Practical Lessons to Help You Implement Change and Achieve Your Goals *By Dr. Misha Galperin*
6 x 9, 192 pp, Quality PB, 978-1-58023-492-4 **$16.99**

Rethinking Synagogues: A New Vocabulary for Congregational Life
By Rabbi Lawrence A. Hoffman, PhD 6 x 9, 240 pp, Quality PB, 978-1-58023-248-7 **$19.99**

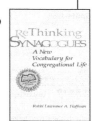

Spiritual Community: The Power to Restore Hope, Commitment and Joy
By Rabbi David A. Teutsch, PhD
5½ x 8½, 144 pp, HC, 978-1-58023-270-8 **$19.99**

Spiritual Boredom: Rediscovering the Wonder of Judaism *By Dr. Erica Brown*
6 x 9, 208 pp, HC, 978-1-58023-405-4 **$21.99**

The Spirituality of Welcoming: How to Transform Your Congregation into a Sacred Community *By Dr. Ron Wolfson* 6 x 9, 224 pp, Quality PB, 978-1-58023-244-9 **$19.99**

Children's Books by Sandy Eisenberg Sasso

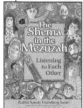

The *Shema* in the Mezuzah: Listening to Each Other
Introduces children ages 3 to 6 to the words of the *Shema* and the custom of putting up the mezuzah. Winner, National Jewish Book Award
9 x 12, 32 pp, Full-color illus., HC, 978-1-58023-506-8 **$18.99**

Adam & Eve's First Sunset: God's New Day
Explores fear and hope, faith and gratitude in ways that will delight kids and adults—inspiring us to bless each of God's days and nights.
9 x 12, 32 pp, Full-color illus., HC, 978-1-58023-177-0 **$17.95** *For ages 4 & up*

Also Available as a Board Book: **Adam and Eve's New Day**
5 x 5, 24 pp, Full-color illus., Board Book, 978-1-59473-205-8 **$7.99** *For ages 1–4*
(A book from SkyLight Paths, Jewish Lights' sister imprint)

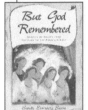

But God Remembered: Stories of Women from Creation to the Promised Land
Four different stories of women—Lilith, Serach, Bityah and the Daughters of Z—teach us important values through their faith and actions.
9 x 12, 32 pp, Full-color illus., Quality PB, 978-1-58023-372-9 **$8.99** *For ages 8 & up*

For Heaven's Sake
Heaven is often found where you least expect it.
9 x 12, 32 pp, Full-color illus., HC, 978-1-58023-054-4 **$16.95** *For ages 4 & up*

God in Between
If you wanted to find God, where would you look? This magical, mythical tale teaches that God can be found where we are: within all of us and the relationships between us. 9 x 12, 32 pp, Full-color illus., HC, 978-1-879045-86-6 **$16.95** *For ages 4 & up*

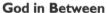

God Said Amen
An inspiring story about hearing the answers to our prayers.
9 x 12, 32 pp, Full-color illus., HC, 978-1-58023-080-3 **$16.95** *For ages 4 & up*

God's Paintbrush: Special 10th Anniversary Edition
Wonderfully interactive, invites children of all faiths and backgrounds to encounter God through moments in their own lives. Provides questions adult and child can explore together. 11 x 8¼, 32 pp, Full-color illus., HC, 978-1-58023-195-4 **$17.95** *For ages 4 & up*

Also Available as a Board Book: **I Am God's Paintbrush**
5 x 5, 24 pp, Full-color illus., Board Book, 978-1-59473-265-2 **$7.99** *For ages 1–4*
(A book from SkyLight Paths, Jewish Lights' sister imprint)

Also Available: **God's Paintbrush Teacher's Guide**
8½ x 11, 32 pp, PB, 978-1-879045-57-6 **$8.95**

God's Paintbrush Celebration Kit
A Spiritual Activity Kit for Teachers and Students of All Faiths, All Backgrounds
9½ x 12, 40 Full-color Activity Sheets & Teacher Folder w/ complete instructions
HC, 978-1-58023-050-6 **$21.95**
8-Student Activity Sheet Pack (40 sheets/5 sessions), 978-1-58023-058-2 **$19.95**

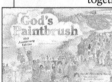

In God's Name
Like an ancient myth in its poetic text and vibrant illustrations, this award-winning modern fable about the search for God's name celebrates the diversity and, at the same time, the unity of all people.
9 x 12, 32 pp, Full-color illus., HC, 978-1-879045-26-2 **$16.99** *For ages 4 & up*

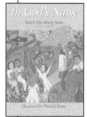

Also Available as a Board Book: **What Is God's Name?**
5 x 5, 24 pp, Full-color illus., Board Book, 978-1-893361-10-2 **$7.99** *For ages 1–4*
(A book from SkyLight Paths, Jewish Lights' sister imprint)

Also Available in Spanish: **El nombre de Dios**
9 x 12, 32 pp, Full-color illus., HC, 978-1-893361-63-8 **$16.95** *For ages 4 & up*

Noah's Wife: The Story of Naamah
9 x 12, 32 pp, Full-color illus., HC, 978-1-58023-134-3 **$16.95** *For ages 4 & up*

Also Available as a Board Book: **Naamah, Noah's Wife**
5 x 5, 24 pp, Full-color illus., Board Book, 978-1-893361-56-0 **$7.95** *For ages 1–4*
(A book from SkyLight Paths, Jewish Lights' sister imprint)

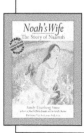

Bar / Bat Mitzvah

The Mitzvah Project Book
Making Mitzvah Part of Your Bar/Bat Mitzvah ... and Your Life
By Liz Suneby and Diane Heiman; Foreword by Rabbi Jeffrey K. Salkin; Preface by Rabbi Sharon Brous
The go-to source for Jewish young adults and their families looking to make the world a better place through good deeds—big or small.
6 x 9, 224 pp, Quality PB Original, 978-1-58023-458-0 **$16.99** *For ages 11–13*

The Bar/Bat Mitzvah Memory Book, 2nd Edition: An Album for Treasuring the Spiritual Celebration
By Rabbi Jeffrey K. Salkin and Nina Salkin
8 x 10, 48 pp, 2-color text, Deluxe HC, ribbon marker, 978-1-58023-263-0 **$19.99**

For Kids—Putting God on Your Guest List, 2nd Edition: How to Claim the Spiritual Meaning of Your Bar or Bat Mitzvah *By Rabbi Jeffrey K. Salkin*
6 x 9, 144 pp, Quality PB, 978-1-58023-308-8 **$15.99** *For ages 11–13*

The Jewish Prophet: Visionary Words from Moses and Miriam to Henrietta Szold and A. J. Heschel *By Rabbi Dr. Michael J. Shire*
6½ x 8½, 128 pp, 123 full-color illus., HC, 978-1-58023-168-8 **$14.95**

Putting God on the Guest List, 3rd Edition: How to Reclaim the Spiritual Meaning of Your Child's Bar or Bat Mitzvah *By Rabbi Jeffrey K. Salkin*
6 x 9, 224 pp, Quality PB, 978-1-58023-222-7 **$16.99**
　　　Teacher's Guide: 8½ x 11, 48 pp, PB, 978-1-58023-226-5 **$8.99**

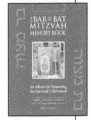
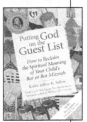

Teens / Young Adults

Text Messages: A Torah Commentary for Teens
Edited by Rabbi Jeffrey K. Salkin
Shows today's teens how each Torah portion contains worlds of meaning for them, for what they are going through in their lives, and how they can shape their Jewish identity as they enter adulthood.
6 x 9, 304 pp (est), HC, 978-1-58023-507-5 **$24.99**

Hannah Senesh: Her Life and Diary, the First Complete Edition
By Hannah Senesh; Foreword by Marge Piercy; Preface by Eitan Senesh; Afterword by Roberta Grossman
6 x 9, 368 pp, b/w photos, Quality PB, 978-1-58023-342-2 **$19.99**

I Am Jewish: Personal Reflections Inspired by the Last Words of Daniel Pearl
Edited by Judea and Ruth Pearl 6 x 9, 304 pp, Deluxe PB w/ flaps, 978-1-58023-259-3 **$19.99**
Download a free copy of the *I Am Jewish Teacher's Guide* at www.jewishlights.com.

The JGirl's Guide: The Young Jewish Woman's Handbook for Coming of Age
By Penina Adelman, Ali Feldman and Shulamit Reinharz
6 x 9, 240 pp, Quality PB, 978-1-58023-215-9 **$14.99** *For ages 11 & up*
　　　Teacher's & Parent's Guide: 8½ x 11, 56 pp, PB, 978-1-58023-225-8 **$8.99**

The JGuy's Guide: The GPS for Jewish Teen Guys
By Rabbi Joseph B. Meszler, Dr. Shulamit Reinharz, Liz Suneby and Diane Heiman
6 x 9, 208 pp, Quality PB Original, 978-1-58023-721-5 **$16.99**
　　　Teacher's Guide: 8½ x 11, 30pp, PB, 978-1-58023-773-4 **$8.99**

Tough Questions Jews Ask, 2nd Edition: A Young Adult's Guide to Building a Jewish Life *By Rabbi Edward Feinstein*
6 x 9, 160 pp, Quality PB, 978-1-58023-454-2 **$16.99** *For ages 11 & up*
　　　Teacher's Guide: 8½ x 11, 72 pp, PB, 978-1-58023-187-9 **$8.95**

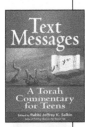
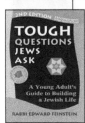

Pre-Teens

Be Like God: God's To-Do List for Kids
By Dr. Ron Wolfson
Encourages kids ages eight through twelve to use their God-given superpowers to find the many ways they can make a difference in the lives of others and find meaning and purpose for their own.
7 x 9, 144 pp, Quality PB, 978-1-58023-510-5 **$15.99** *For ages 8–12*

The Book of Miracles: A Young Person's Guide to Jewish Spiritual Awareness
By Lawrence Kushner, with all-new illustrations by the author.
6 x 9, 96 pp, 2-color illus., HC, 978-1-879045-78-1 **$16.95** *For ages 9–13*

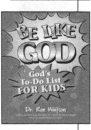

Children's Books

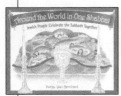

Around the World in One Shabbat
Jewish People Celebrate the Sabbath Together
By Durga Yael Bernhard
Takes your child on a colorful adventure to share the many ways Jewish people celebrate Shabbat around the world.
11 x 8½, 32 pp, Full-color illus., HC, 978-1-58023-433-7 **$18.99** *For ages 3–6*

It's a ... It's a ... It's a Mitzvah
By Liz Suneby and Diane Heiman; Full-color Illus. by Laurel Molk
Join Mitzvah Meerkat and friends as they introduce children to the everyday kindnesses that mark the beginning of a Jewish journey and a lifetime commitment to *tikkun olam* (repairing the world). 9 x 12, 32 pp, Full-color illus., HC, 978-1-58023-509-9 **$18.99** *For ages 3–6*

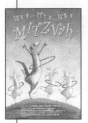

What You Will See Inside a Synagogue
By Rabbi Lawrence A. Hoffman, PhD, and Dr. Ron Wolfson; Full-color photos by Bill Aron
A colorful, fun-to-read introduction that explains the ways and whys of Jewish worship and religious life. 8½ x 10½, 32 pp, Full-color photos, Quality PB, 978-1-59473-256-0 **$8.99** *For ages 6 & up*
(A book from SkyLight Paths, Jewish Lights' sister imprint)

Because Nothing Looks Like God
By Lawrence Kushner and Karen Kushner
Real-life examples of happiness and sadness—from goodnight stories, to the hope and fear felt the first time at bat, to the closing moments of someone's life—invite parents and children to explore, together, the questions we all have about God, no matter what our age. 11 x 8½, 32 pp, Full-color illus., HC, 978-1-58023-092-6 **$18.99** *For ages 4 & up*

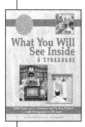

The Book of Miracles: A Young Person's Guide to Jewish Spiritual Awareness
Written and illus. by Lawrence Kushner
Easy-to-read, imaginatively illustrated book encourages kids' awareness of their own spirituality. Revealing the essence of Judaism in a language they can understand and enjoy. 6 x 9, 96 pp, 2-color illus., HC, 978-1-879045-78-1 **$16.95** *For ages 9–13*

In God's Hands   *By Lawrence Kushner and Gary Schmidt*
Brings new life to a traditional Jewish folktale, reminding parents and kids of all faiths and all backgrounds that each of us has the power to make the world a better place—working ordinary miracles with our everyday deeds.
9 x 12, 32 pp, Full-color illus., HC, 978-1-58023-224-1 **$16.99** *For ages 5 & up*

In Our Image: God's First Creatures
By Nancy Sohn Swartz
A playful new twist to the Genesis story, God asks all of nature to offer gifts to humankind—with a promise that the humans would care for creation in return. 9 x 12, 32 pp, Full-color illus., HC, 978-1-879045-99-6 **$16.95** *For ages 4 & up*
Animated app available on Apple App Store and The Google Play Marketplace **$9.99**

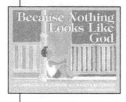

The Jewish Family Fun Book, 2nd Ed.
Holiday Projects, Everyday Activities, and Travel Ideas with Jewish Themes
By Danielle Dardashti and Roni Sarig
The complete sourcebook for families wanting to put a new spin on activities for Jewish holidays, holy days and the everyday. It offers dozens of easy-to-do activities that bring Jewish tradition to life for kids of all ages.
6 x 9, 304 pp, w/ 70+ b/w illus., Quality PB, 978-1-58023-333-0 **$18.99**

What Makes Someone a Jew?   *By Lauren Seidman*
Reflects the changing face of American Judaism. Helps preschoolers and young readers (ages 3–6) understand that you don't have to look a certain way to be Jewish.
10 x 8½, 32 pp, Full-color photos, Quality PB, 978-1-58023-321-7 **$8.99** *For ages 3–6*

When a Grandparent Dies: A Kid's Own Remembering Workbook for
Dealing with Shiva and the Year Beyond   *By Nechama Liss-Levinson*
8 x 10, 48 pp, 2-color text, HC, 978-1-879045-44-6 **$15.95** *For ages 7–13*

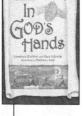

Spirituality / Crafts

Jewish Threads: A Hands-On Guide to Stitching Spiritual Intention into Jewish Fabric Crafts *By Diana Drew with Robert Grayson*
Learn how to make your own Jewish fabric crafts with spiritual intention—a journey of creativity, imagination and inspiration. Thirty projects.
7 x 9, 288 pp, 8-page color insert, b/w illus., Quality PB Original, 978-1-58023-442-9 **$19.99**

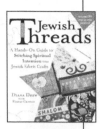

Beading—The Creative Spirit: Finding Your Sacred Center through the Art of Beadwork *By Wendy Ellsworth*
Invites you on a spiritual pilgrimage into the kaleidoscope world of glass and color.
7 x 9, 240 pp, 8-page full-color insert, b/w photos and diagrams, Quality PB, 978-1-59473-267-6 **$18.99***

Contemplative Crochet: A Hands-On Guide for Interlocking Faith and Craft *By Cindy Crandall-Frazier; Foreword by Linda Skolnik*
Will take you on a path deeper into your crocheting and your spiritual awareness.
7 x 9, 208 pp, b/w photos, Quality PB, 978-1-59473-238-6 **$16.99***

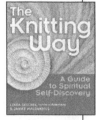

The Knitting Way: A Guide to Spiritual Self-Discovery
By Linda Skolnik and Janice MacDaniels
Shows how to use knitting to strengthen your spiritual self.
7 x 9, 240 pp, b/w photos, Quality PB, 978-1-59473-079-5 **$16.99***

The Painting Path: Embodying Spiritual Discovery through Yoga, Brush and Color *By Linda Novick; Foreword by Richard Segalman*
Explores the divine connection you can experience through art.
7 x 9, 208 pp, 8-page full-color insert, b/w photos, Quality PB, 978-1-59473-226-3 **$18.99***

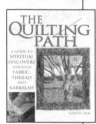

The Quilting Path: A Guide to Spiritual Self-Discovery through Fabric, Thread and Kabbalah *By Louise Silk* Explores how to cultivate personal growth through quilt making. 7 x 9, 192 pp, b/w photos, Quality PB, 978-1-59473-206-5 **$16.99***

Travel / History

Israel—A Spiritual Travel Guide, 2nd Edition: A Companion for the Modern Jewish Pilgrim *By Rabbi Lawrence A. Hoffman, PhD*
Helps today's pilgrim tap into the deep spiritual meaning of the ancient—and modern—sites of the Holy Land.
4¾ x 10, 256 pp, Illus., Quality PB, 978-1-58023-261-6 **$18.99**
Also Available: **The Israel Mission Leader's Guide** 5½ x 8½, 16 pp, PB, 978-1-58023-085-8 **$4.95**

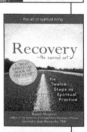

On the Chocolate Trail: A Delicious Adventure Connecting Jews, Religions, History, Travel, Rituals and Recipes to the Magic of Cacao
By Rabbi Deborah R. Prinz
Take a delectable journey through the religious history of chocolate—a real treat!
6 x 9, 272 pp w/ 20+ b/w photographs, Quality PB, 978-1-58023-487-0 **$18.99**

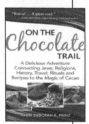

Twelve Steps

Recovery—The Sacred Art: The Twelve Steps as Spiritual Practice
By Rami Shapiro; Foreword by Joan Borysenko, PhD
Draws on insights and practices of different religious traditions to help you move more deeply into the universal spirituality of the Twelve Step system.
5½ x 8½, 240 pp, Quality PB Original, 978-1-59473-259-1 **$16.99***

100 Blessings Every Day: Daily Twelve Step Recovery Affirmations, Exercises for Personal Growth & Renewal Reflecting Seasons of the Jewish Year *By Rabbi Kerry M. Olitzky; Foreword by Rabbi Neil Gillman, PhD* 4¼ x 6¼, 432 pp, Quality PB, 978-1-879045-30-9 **$16.99**

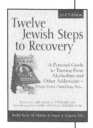

Recovery from Codependence: A Jewish Twelve Steps Guide to Healing Your Soul
By Rabbi Kerry M. Olitzky 6 x 9, 160 pp, Quality PB, 978-1-879045-32-3 **$13.95**

Twelve Jewish Steps to Recovery, 2nd Edition: A Personal Guide to Turning from Alcoholism & Other Addictions—Drugs, Food, Gambling, Sex…
By Rabbi Kerry M. Olitzky and Stuart A. Copans, MD; Preface by Abraham J. Twerski, MD
6 x 9, 160 pp, Quality PB, 978-1-58023-409-2 **$16.99**

A book from SkyLight Paths, Jewish Lights' sister imprint

Ecology / Environment

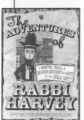

A Wild Faith: Jewish Ways into Wilderness, Wilderness Ways into Judaism
By Rabbi Mike Comins; Foreword by Nigel Savage 6 x 9, 240 pp, Quality PB, 978-1-58023-316-3 **$16.99**

Ecology & the Jewish Spirit: Where Nature & the Sacred Meet
Edited by Ellen Bernstein 6 x 9, 288 pp, Quality PB, 978-1-58023-082-7 **$18.99**

Torah of the Earth: Exploring 4,000 Years of Ecology in Jewish Thought
Vol. 1: Biblical Israel & Rabbinic Judaism; Vol. 2: Zionism & Eco-Judaism
Edited by Rabbi Arthur Waskow Vol. 1: 6 x 9, 272 pp, Quality PB, 978-1-58023-086-5 **$19.95**
Vol. 2: 6 x 9, 336 pp, Quality PB, 978-1-58023-087-2 **$19.95**

The Way Into Judaism and the Environment *By Jeremy Benstein, PhD*
6 x 9, 288 pp, Quality PB, 978-1-58023-368-2 **$18.99**; HC, 978-1-58023-268-5 **$24.99**

Graphic Novels / Graphic History

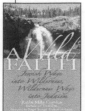

The Adventures of Rabbi Harvey: A Graphic Novel of Jewish Wisdom and Wit in the
Wild West *By Steve Sheinkin* 6 x 9, 144 pp, Full-color illus., Quality PB, 978-1-58023-310-1 **$16.99**

Rabbi Harvey Rides Again: A Graphic Novel of Jewish Folktales Let Loose in the
Wild West *By Steve Sheinkin* 6 x 9, 144 pp, Full-color illus., Quality PB, 978-1-58023-347-7 **$16.99**

Rabbi Harvey vs. the Wisdom Kid: A Graphic Novel of Dueling Jewish Folktales in
the Wild West *By Steve Sheinkin*
6 x 9, 144 pp, Full-color illus., Quality PB, 978-1-58023-422-1 **$16.99**

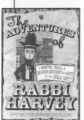

The Story of the Jews: A 4,000-Year Adventure—A Graphic History Book
By Stan Mack 6 x 9, 288 pp, Illus., Quality PB, 978-1-58023-155-8 **$16.99**

Grief / Healing

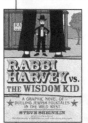

Judaism and Health: A Handbook of Practical, Professional and Scholarly
Resources *Edited by Jeff Levin, PhD, MPH, and Michele F. Prince, LCSW, MAJCS*
Foreword by Rabbi Elliot N. Dorff, PhD
Explores the expressions of health in the form of overviews of research studies,
first-person narratives and advice. 6 x 9, 448 pp, HC, 978-1-58023-714-7 **$50.00**

Facing Illness, Finding God: How Judaism Can Help You and Caregivers Cope
When Body or Spirit Fails *By Rabbi Joseph B. Meszler*
6 x 9, 208 pp, Quality PB, 978-1-58023-423-8 **$16.99**

Grief in Our Seasons: A Mourner's Kaddish Companion *By Rabbi Kerry M. Olitzky*
4½ x 6½, 448 pp, Quality PB, 978-1-879045-55-2 **$15.95**

Healing and the Jewish Imagination: Spiritual and Practical Perspectives on
Judaism and Health *Edited by Rabbi William Cutter, PhD*
6 x 9, 240 pp, Quality PB, 978-1-58023-373-6 **$19.99**

Healing from Despair: Choosing Wholeness in a Broken World
By Rabbi Elie Kaplan Spitz with Erica Shapiro Taylor; Foreword by Abraham J. Twerski, MD
5½ x 8½, 208 pp, Quality PB, 978-1-58023-436-8 **$16.99**

Healing of Soul, Healing of Body: Spiritual Leaders Unfold the Strength & Solace
in Psalms *Edited by Rabbi Simkha Y. Weintraub, LCSW*
6 x 9, 128 pp, 2-color illus. text, Quality PB, 978-1-879045-31-6 **$16.99**

Midrash & Medicine: Healing Body and Soul in the Jewish Interpretive Tradition
Edited by Rabbi William Cutter, PhD; Foreword by Michele F. Prince, LCSW, MAJCS
6 x 9, 352 pp, Quality PB, 978-1-58023-484-9 **$21.99**

Mourning & Mitzvah, 2nd Edition: A Guided Journal for Walking the Mourner's
Path through Grief to Healing *By Rabbi Anne Brener, LCSW*
7½ x 9, 304 pp, Quality PB, 978-1-58023-113-8 **$19.99**

Tears of Sorrow, Seeds of Hope, 2nd Edition: A Jewish Spiritual Companion
for Infertility and Pregnancy Loss *By Rabbi Nina Beth Cardin*
6 x 9, 208 pp, Quality PB, 978-1-58023-233-3 **$18.99**

A Time to Mourn, a Time to Comfort, 2nd Edition: A Guide to Jewish
Bereavement *By Dr. Ron Wolfson; Foreword by Rabbi David J. Wolpe*
7 x 9, 384 pp, Quality PB, 978-1-58023-253-1 **$21.99**

When a Grandparent Dies: A Kid's Own Remembering Workbook for Dealing
with Shiva and the Year Beyond *By Nechama Liss-Levinson, PhD*
8 x 10, 48 pp, 2-color text, HC, 978-1-879045-44-6 **$15.95** *For ages 7–13*

Theology / Philosophy / The Way Into... Series

The Way Into... series offers an accessible and highly usable "guided tour" of the Jewish faith, people, history and beliefs—in total, an introduction to Judaism that will enable you to understand and interact with the sacred texts of the Jewish tradition. Each volume is written by a leading contemporary scholar and teacher, and explores one key aspect of Judaism. The Way Into... series enables all readers to achieve a real sense of Jewish cultural literacy through guided study.

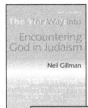

The Way Into Encountering God in Judaism
By Rabbi Neil Gillman, PhD
For everyone who wants to understand how Jews have encountered God throughout history and today.
6 x 9, 240 pp, Quality PB, 978-1-58023-199-2 **$18.99**; HC, 978-1-58023-025-4 **$21.95**
Also Available: **The Jewish Approach to God:** A Brief Introduction for Christians
  By Rabbi Neil Gillman, PhD
  5½ x 8½, 192 pp, Quality PB, 978-1-58023-190-9 **$16.95**

The Way Into Jewish Mystical Tradition
By Rabbi Lawrence Kushner
Allows readers to interact directly with the sacred mystical texts of the Jewish tradition. An accessible introduction to the concepts of Jewish mysticism, their religious and spiritual significance, and how they relate to life today.
6 x 9, 224 pp, Quality PB, 978-1-58023-200-5 **$18.99**

The Way Into Jewish Prayer
By Rabbi Lawrence A. Hoffman, PhD
Opens the door to 3,000 years of Jewish prayer, making anyone feel at home in the Jewish way of communicating with God.
6 x 9, 208 pp, Quality PB, 978-1-58023-201-2 **$18.99**

The Way Into Jewish Prayer Teacher's Guide
  By Rabbi Jennifer Ossakow Goldsmith
  8½ x 11, 42 pp, PB, 978-1-58023-345-3 **$8.99**
  Download a free copy at www.jewishlights.com.

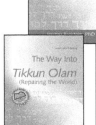

The Way Into Judaism and the Environment
By Jeremy Benstein, PhD
Explores the ways in which Judaism contributes to contemporary social-environmental issues, the extent to which Judaism is part of the problem and how it can be part of the solution.
6 x 9, 288 pp, Quality PB, 978-1-58023-368-2 **$18.99**; HC, 978-1-58023-268-5 **$24.99**

The Way Into *Tikkun Olam* (Repairing the World)
By Rabbi Elliot N. Dorff, PhD
An accessible introduction to the Jewish concept of the individual's responsibility to care for others and repair the world.
6 x 9, 304 pp, Quality PB, 978-1-58023-328-6 **$18.99**

The Way Into Torah
By Rabbi Norman J. Cohen, PhD
Helps guide you in the exploration of the origins and development of Torah, explains why it should be studied and how to do it.
6 x 9, 176 pp, Quality PB, 978-1-58023-198-5 **$16.99**

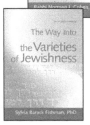

The Way Into the Varieties of Jewishness
By Sylvia Barack Fishman, PhD
Explores the religious and historical understanding of what it has meant to be Jewish from ancient times to the present controversy over "Who is a Jew?"
6 x 9, 288 pp, Quality PB, 978-1-58023-367-5 **$18.99**; HC, 978-1-58023-030-8 **$24.99**

Theology / Philosophy

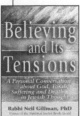

Believing and Its Tensions: A Personal Conversation about God, Torah, Suffering and Death in Jewish Thought
By Rabbi Neil Gillman, PhD
Explores the changing nature of belief and the complexities of reconciling the intellectual, emotional and moral questions of Gillman's own searching mind and soul.
5½ x 8½, 144 pp, HC, 978-1-58023-669-0 **$19.99**

God of Becoming and Relationship: The Dynamic Nature of Process Theology   *By Rabbi Bradley Shavit Artson, DHL*
Explains how Process Theology breaks us free from the strictures of ancient Greek and medieval European philosophy, allowing us to see all creation as related patterns of energy through which we connect to everything.
6 x 9, 208 pp, HC, 978-1-58023-713-0 **$24.99**

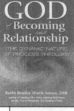

The Other Talmud—The *Yerushalmi*: Unlocking the Secrets of *The Talmud of Israel* for Judaism Today   *By Rabbi Judith Z. Abrams, PhD*
A fascinating—and stimulating—look at "the other Talmud" and the possibilities for Jewish life reflected there.   6 x 9, 256 pp, HC, 978-1-58023-463-4 **$24.99**

The Way of Man: According to Hasidic Teaching
By Martin Buber; New Translation and Introduction by Rabbi Bernard H. Mehlman and Dr. Gabriel E. Padawer; Foreword by Paul Mendes-Flohr
An accessible and engaging new translation of Buber's classic work—*available as an e-book only.*   E-book, 978-1-58023-601-0 Digital List Price **$14.99**

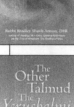

The Death of Death: Resurrection and Immortality in Jewish Thought
By Rabbi Neil Gillman, PhD 6 x 9, 336 pp, Quality PB, 978-1-58023-081-0 **$18.95**

Doing Jewish Theology: God, Torah & Israel in Modern Judaism *By Rabbi Neil Gillman, PhD*
6 x 9, 304 pp, Quality PB, 978-1-58023-439-9 **$18.99**; HC, 978-1-58023-322-4 **$24.99**

From Defender to Critic: The Search for a New Jewish Self
By Dr. David Hartman 6 x 9, 336 pp, HC, 978-1-58023-515-0 **$35.00**

The God Who Hates Lies: Confronting & Rethinking Jewish Tradition
By Dr. David Hartman with Charlie Buckholtz 6 x 9, 208 pp, Quality PB, 978-1-58023-790-1 **$19.99**

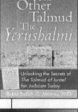

A Heart of Many Rooms: Celebrating the Many Voices within Judaism
By Dr. David Hartman 6 x 9, 352 pp, Quality PB, 978-1-58023-156-5 **$19.95**

Jewish Theology in Our Time: A New Generation Explores the Foundations and Future of Jewish Belief   *Edited by Rabbi Elliot J. Cosgrove, PhD; Foreword by Rabbi David J. Wolpe; Preface by Rabbi Carole B. Balin, PhD* 6 x 9, 240 pp, Quality PB, 978-1-58023-630-1, **$19.99**; HC, 978-1-58023-413-9 **$24.99**

Maimonides—Essential Teachings on Jewish Faith & Ethics: The Book of Knowledge & the Thirteen Principles of Faith—Annotated & Explained
Translation and Annotation by Rabbi Marc D. Angel, PhD
5½ x 8½, 224 pp, Quality PB Original, 978-1-59473-311-6 **$18.99***

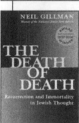

Maimonides, Spinoza and Us: Toward an Intellectually Vibrant Judaism
By Rabbi Marc D. Angel, PhD 6 x 9, 224 pp, HC, 978-1-58023-411-5 **$24.99**

Our Religious Brains: What Cognitive Science Reveals about Belief, Morality, Community and Our Relationship with God
By Rabbi Ralph D. Mecklenburger; Foreword by Dr. Howard Kelfer; Preface by Dr. Neil Gillman
6 x 9, 224 pp, HC, 978-1-58023-508-2 **$24.99**

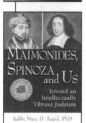

Your Word Is Fire: The Hasidic Masters on Contemplative Prayer
Edited and translated by Rabbi Arthur Green, PhD, and Barry W. Holtz
6 x 9, 160 pp, Quality PB, 978-1-879045-25-5 **$16.99**

I Am Jewish
Personal Reflections Inspired by the Last Words of Daniel Pearl
Almost 150 Jews—both famous and not—from all walks of life, from all around the world, write about many aspects of their Judaism.
   Edited by Judea and Ruth Pearl   6 x 9, 304 pp, Deluxe PB w/ flaps, 978-1-58023-259-3 **$19.99**
Download a free copy of the *I Am Jewish Teacher's Guide* at www.jewishlights.com.

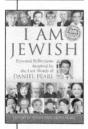

*A book from SkyLight Paths, Jewish Lights' sister imprint

Inspiration

Into the Fullness of the Void: A Spiritual Autobiography *By Dov Elbaum*
The spiritual autobiography of one of Israel's leading cultural figures that provides insights and guidance for all of us. 6 x 9, 304 pp, Quality PB Original, 978-1-58023-715-4 **$18.99**

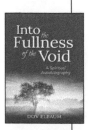

Saying No and Letting Go: Jewish Wisdom on Making Room for What Matters Most
By Rabbi Edwin Goldberg, DHL; Foreword by Rabbi Naomi Levy
Taps into timeless Jewish wisdom that teaches how to "hold on tightly" to the things that matter most while learning to "let go lightly" of the demands and worries that do not ultimately matter. 6 x 9, 192 pp, Quality PB, 978-1-58023-670-6 **$16.99**

The Bridge to Forgiveness: Stories and Prayers for Finding God and Restoring Wholeness *By Rabbi Karyn D. Kedar* 6 x 9, 176 pp, Quality PB, 978-1-58023-451-1 **$16.99**

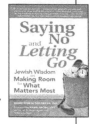

The Empty Chair: Finding Hope and Joy—Timeless Wisdom from a Hasidic Master, Rebbe Nachman of Breslov *Adapted by Moshe Mykoff and the Breslov Research Institute*
4 x 6, 128 pp, Deluxe PB w/ flaps, 978-1-879045-67-5 **$9.99**

A Formula for Proper Living: Practical Lessons from Life and Torah
By Rabbi Abraham J. Twerski, MD 6 x 9, 144 pp, HC, 978-1-58023-402-3 **$19.99**

The Gentle Weapon: Prayers for Everyday and Not-So-Everyday Moments—Timeless Wisdom from the Teachings of the Hasidic Master, Rebbe Nachman of Breslov
Adapted by Moshe Mykoff and S. C. Mizrahi, together with the Breslov Research Institute
4 x 6, 144 pp, Deluxe PB w/ flaps, 978-1-58023-022-3 **$9.99**

The God Upgrade: Finding Your 21st-Century Spirituality in Judaism's 5,000-Year-Old Tradition *By Rabbi Jamie Korngold; Foreword by Rabbi Harold M. Schulweis*
6 x 9, 176 pp, Quality PB, 978-1-58023-443-6 **$15.99**

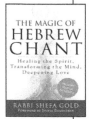

God Whispers: Stories of the Soul, Lessons of the Heart *By Rabbi Karyn D. Kedar*
6 x 9, 176 pp, Quality PB, 978-1-58023-088-9 **$15.95**

God's To-Do List: 103 Ways to Be an Angel and Do God's Work on Earth
By Dr. Ron Wolfson 6 x 9, 144 pp, Quality PB, 978-1-58023-301-9 **$16.99**

Happiness and the Human Spirit: The Spirituality of Becoming the Best You Can Be
By Rabbi Abraham J. Twerski, MD
6 x 9, 176 pp, Quality PB, 978-1-58023-404-7 **$16.99**; HC, 978-1-58023-343-9 **$19.99**

Life's Daily Blessings: Inspiring Reflections on Gratitude and Joy for Every Day, Based on Jewish Wisdom *By Rabbi Kerry M. Olitzky* 4½ x 6½, 368 pp, Quality PB, 978-1-58023-396-5 **$16.99**

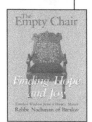

The Magic of Hebrew Chant: Healing the Spirit, Transforming the Mind, Deepening Love *By Rabbi Shefa Gold; Foreword by Sylvia Boorstein*
6 x 9, 352 pp, Quality PB, 978-1-58023-671-3 **$24.99**

Restful Reflections: Nighttime Inspiration to Calm the Soul, Based on Jewish Wisdom
By Rabbi Kerry M. Olitzky and Rabbi Lori Forman-Jacobi 5 x 8, 352 pp, Quality PB, 978-1-58023-091-9 **$16.99**

Sacred Intentions: Morning Inspiration to Strengthen the Spirit, Based on Jewish Wisdom
By Rabbi Kerry M. Olitzky and Rabbi Lori Forman-Jacobi 4½ x 6½, 448 pp, Quality PB, 978-1-58023-061-2 **$16.99**

The Seven Questions You're Asked in Heaven: Reviewing and Renewing Your Life on Earth *By Dr. Ron Wolfson* 6 x 9, 176 pp, Quality PB, 978-1-58023-407-8 **$16.99**

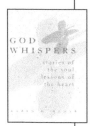

Kabbalah / Mysticism

Ehyeh: A Kabbalah for Tomorrow
By Rabbi Arthur Green, PhD 6 x 9, 224 pp, Quality PB, 978-1-58023-213-5 **$18.99**

The Gift of Kabbalah: Discovering the Secrets of Heaven, Renewing Your Life on Earth
By Tamar Frankiel, PhD 6 x 9, 256 pp, Quality PB, 978-1-58023-141-1 **$16.95**

Jewish Mysticism and the Spiritual Life: Classical Texts, Contemporary Reflections *Edited by Dr. Lawrence Fine, Dr. Eitan Fishbane and Rabbi Or N. Rose*
6 x 9, 256 pp, HC, 978-1-58023-434-4 **$24.99**; Quality PB, 978-1-58023-719-2 **$18.99**

Seek My Face: A Jewish Mystical Theology *By Rabbi Arthur Green, PhD*
6 x 9, 304 pp, Quality PB, 978-1-58023-130-5 **$19.95**

Zohar: Annotated & Explained *Translation & Annotation by Dr. Daniel C. Matt; Foreword by Andrew Harvey* 5½ x 8½, 176 pp, Quality PB, 978-1-893361-51-5 **$16.99**
(A book from SkyLight Paths, Jewish Lights' sister imprint)

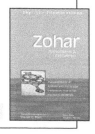

See also *The Way Into Jewish Mystical Tradition* in The Way Into... Series.

Spirituality / Prayer

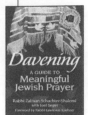

Davening: A Guide to Meaningful Jewish Prayer
By Rabbi Zalman Schachter-Shalomi with Joel Segel; Foreword by Rabbi Lawrence Kushner
A fresh approach to prayer for all who wish to appreciate the power of prayer's poetry, song and ritual, and to join the age-old conversation that Jews have had with God. 6 x 9, 240 pp, Quality PB, 978-1-58023-627-0 **$18.99**

Jewish Men Pray: Words of Yearning, Praise, Petition, Gratitude and Wonder from Traditional and Contemporary Sources
Edited by Rabbi Kerry M. Olitzky and Stuart M. Matlins; Foreword by Rabbi Bradley Shavit Artson, DHL
A celebration of Jewish men's voices in prayer—to strengthen, heal, comfort, and inspire—from the ancient world up to our own day.
5 x 7¼, 400 pp, HC, 978-1-58023-628-7 **$19.99**

Making Prayer Real: Leading Jewish Spiritual Voices on Why Prayer Is Difficult and What to Do about It *By Rabbi Mike Comins* 6 x 9, 320 pp, Quality PB, 978-1-58023-417-7 **$18.99**

Witnesses to the One: The Spiritual History of the *Sh'ma*
By Rabbi Joseph B. Meszler; Foreword by Rabbi Elyse Goldstein
6 x 9, 176 pp, Quality PB, 978-1-58023-400-9 **$16.99**; HC, 978-1-58023-309-5 **$19.99**

My People's Prayer Book Series: Traditional Prayers, Modern Commentaries *Edited by Rabbi Lawrence A. Hoffman, PhD*
Provides diverse and exciting commentary to the traditional liturgy. Will help you find new wisdom in Jewish prayer, and bring liturgy into your life. Each book includes Hebrew text, modern translations and commentaries from all perspectives of the Jewish world.

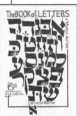

Vol. 1—The *Sh'ma* and Its Blessings
7 x 10, 168 pp, HC, 978-1-879045-79-8 **$29.99**
Vol. 2—The *Amidah* 7 x 10, 240 pp, HC, 978-1-879045-80-4 **$24.95**
Vol. 3—*P'sukei D'zimrah* (Morning Psalms)
7 x 10, 240 pp, HC, 978-1-879045-81-1 **$29.99**
Vol. 4—*Seder K'riat Hatorah* (The Torah Service)
7 x 10, 264 pp, HC, 978-1-879045-82-8 **$29.99**
Vol. 5—*Birkhot Hashachar* (Morning Blessings)
7 x 10, 240 pp, HC, 978-1-879045-83-5 **$24.95**
Vol. 6—*Tachanun* and Concluding Prayers
7 x 10, 240 pp, HC, 978-1-879045-84-2 **$24.95**
Vol. 7—Shabbat at Home 7 x 10, 240 pp, HC, 978-1-879045-85-9 **$24.95**
Vol. 8—*Kabbalat Shabbat* (Welcoming Shabbat in the Synagogue)
7 x 10, 240 pp, HC, 978-1-58023-121-3 **$24.99**
Vol. 9—Welcoming the Night: *Minchah* and *Ma'ariv* (Afternoon and Evening Prayer) 7 x 10, 272 pp, HC, 978-1-58023-262-3 **$24.99**
Vol. 10—Shabbat Morning: *Shacharit* and *Musaf* (Morning and Additional Services) 7 x 10, 240 pp, HC, 978-1-58023-240-1 **$29.99**

Spirituality / Lawrence Kushner

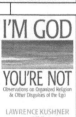

I'm God; You're Not: Observations on Organized Religion & Other Disguises of the Ego
6 x 9, 256 pp, Quality PB, 978-1-58023-513-6 **$18.99**; HC, 978-1-58023-441-2 **$21.99**

The Book of Letters: A Mystical Hebrew Alphabet
Popular HC Edition, 6 x 9, 80 pp, 2-color text, 978-1-879045-00-2 **$24.95**
Collector's Limited Edition, 9 x 12, 80 pp, gold-foil-embossed pages, w/ limited-edition silkscreened print, 978-1-879045-04-0 **$349.00**

The Book of Miracles: A Young Person's Guide to Jewish Spiritual Awareness
6 x 9, 96 pp, 2-color illus., HC, 978-1-879045-78-1 **$16.95** *For ages 9–13*

God Was in This Place & I, i Did Not Know: Finding Self, Spirituality and Ultimate Meaning 6 x 9, 192 pp, Quality PB, 978-1-879045-33-0 **$16.95**

Honey from the Rock: An Introduction to Jewish Mysticism
6 x 9, 176 pp, Quality PB, 978-1-58023-073-5 **$18.99**

Invisible Lines of Connection: Sacred Stories of the Ordinary
5½ x 8½, 160 pp, Quality PB, 978-1-879045-98-9 **$16.99**

The Way Into Jewish Mystical Tradition
6 x 9, 224 pp, Quality PB, 978-1-58023-200-5 **$18.99**; HC, 978-1-58023-029-2 **$21.95**

Spirituality

Amazing Chesed: Living a Grace-Filled Judaism
By Rabbi Rami Shapiro Drawing from ancient and contemporary, traditional and non-traditional Jewish wisdom, reclaims the idea of grace in Judaism.
6 x 9, 176 pp, Quality PB, 978-1-58023-624-9 **$16.99**

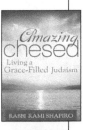

Jewish with Feeling: A Guide to Meaningful Jewish Practice
By Rabbi Zalman Schachter-Shalomi with Joel Segel
Takes off from basic questions like "Why be Jewish?" and whether the word God still speaks to us today and lays out a vision for a whole-person Judaism.
5½ x 8½, 288 pp, Quality PB, 978-1-58023-691-1 **$19.99**

Perennial Wisdom for the Spiritually Independent: Sacred Teachings—Annotated & Explained *Annotation by Rami Shapiro; Foreword by Richard Rohr*
Weaves sacred texts and teachings from the world's major religions into a coherent exploration of the five core questions at the heart of every religion's search.
5½ x 8½, 336 pp, Quality PB Original, 978-1-59473-515-8 **$16.99**

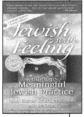

Aleph-Bet Yoga: Embodying the Hebrew Letters for Physical and Spiritual Well-Being
By Steven A. Rapp; Foreword by Tamar Frankiel, PhD, and Judy Greenfeld; Preface by Hart Lazer
7 x 10, 128 pp, b/w photos, Quality PB, Lay-flat binding, 978-1-58023-162-6 **$16.95**

A Book of Life: Embracing Judaism as a Spiritual Practice
By Rabbi Michael Strassfeld 6 x 9, 544 pp, Quality PB, 978-1-58023-247-0 **$19.99**

Bringing the Psalms to Life: How to Understand and Use the Book of Psalms
By Rabbi Daniel F. Polish, PhD 6 x 9, 208 pp, Quality PB, 978-1-58023-157-2 **$16.95**

Does the Soul Survive? A Jewish Journey to Belief in Afterlife, Past Lives & Living with Purpose *By Rabbi Elie Kaplan Spitz; Foreword by Brian L. Weiss, MD*
6 x 9, 288 pp, Quality PB, 978-1-58023-165-7 **$18.99**

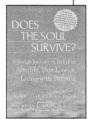

Entering the Temple of Dreams: Jewish Prayers, Movements and Meditations for the End of the Day *By Tamar Frankiel, PhD, and Judy Greenfeld*
7 x 10, 192 pp, illus., Quality PB, 978-1-58023-079-7 **$16.95**

First Steps to a New Jewish Spirit: Reb Zalman's Guide to Recapturing the Intimacy & Ecstasy in Your Relationship with God *By Rabbi Zalman M. Schachter-Shalomi with Donald Gropman* 6 x 9, 144 pp, Quality PB, 978-1-58023-182-4 **$16.95**

Foundations of Sephardic Spirituality: The Inner Life of Jews of the Ottoman Empire
By Rabbi Marc D. Angel, PhD 6 x 9, 224 pp, Quality PB, 978-1-58023-341-5 **$18.99**

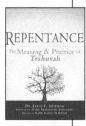

God & the Big Bang: Discovering Harmony between Science & Spirituality
By Dr. Daniel C. Matt 6 x 9, 216 pp, Quality PB, 978-1-879045-89-7 **$18.99**

God in Our Relationships: Spirituality between People from the Teachings of Martin Buber *By Rabbi Dennis S. Ross* 5½ x 8½, 160 pp, Quality PB, 978-1-58023-147-3 **$16.95**

The Jewish Lights Spirituality Handbook: A Guide to Understanding, Exploring & Living a Spiritual Life *Edited by Stuart M. Matlins*
6 x 9, 456 pp, Quality PB, 978-1-58023-093-3 **$19.99**

Judaism, Physics and God: Searching for Sacred Metaphors in a Post-Einstein World
By Rabbi David W. Nelson 6 x 9, 352 pp, Quality PB, inc. reader's discussion guide,
978-1-58023-306-4 **$18.99**; HC, 352 pp, 978-1-58023-252-4 **$24.99**

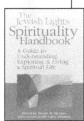

Meaning & Mitzvah: Daily Practices for Reclaiming Judaism through Prayer, God, Torah, Hebrew, Mitzvot and Peoplehood *By Rabbi Goldie Milgram*
7 x 9, 336 pp, Quality PB, 978-1-58023-256-2 **$19.99**

Repentance: The Meaning and Practice of Teshuvah
By Dr. Louis E. Newman; Foreword by Rabbi Harold M. Schulweis; Preface by Rabbi Karyn D. Kedar
6 x 9, 256 pp, HC, 978-1-58023-426-9 **$24.99** Quality PB, 978-1-58023-718-5 **$18.99**

The Sabbath Soul: Mystical Reflections on the Transformative Power of Holy Time
Selection, Translation and Commentary by Eitan Fishbane, PhD
6 x 9, 208 pp, Quality PB, 978-1-58023-459-7 **$18.99**

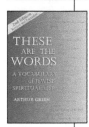

Tanya, the Masterpiece of Hasidic Wisdom: Selections Annotated & Explained
Translation & Annotation by Rabbi Rami Shapiro; Foreword by Rabbi Zalman M. Schachter-Shalomi
5½ x 8½, 240 pp, Quality PB, 978-1-59473-275-1 **$16.99**

These Are the Words, 2nd Edition: A Vocabulary of Jewish Spiritual Life
By Rabbi Arthur Green, PhD 6 x 9, 320 pp, Quality PB, 978-1-58023-494-8 **$19.99**

Social Justice

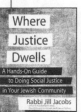

Where Justice Dwells
A Hands-On Guide to Doing Social Justice in Your Jewish Community
By Rabbi Jill Jacobs; Foreword by Rabbi David Saperstein
Provides ways to envision and act on your own ideals of social justice.
7 x 9, 288 pp, Quality PB Original, 978-1-58023-453-5 **$24.99**

There Shall Be No Needy
Pursuing Social Justice through Jewish Law and Tradition
By Rabbi Jill Jacobs; Foreword by Rabbi Elliot N. Dorff, PhD; Preface by Simon Greer
Confronts the most pressing issues of twenty-first-century America from a deeply
Jewish perspective. 6 x 9, 288 pp, Quality PB, 978-1-58023-425-2 **$16.99**

There Shall Be No Needy Teacher's Guide 8½ x 11, 56 pp, PB, 978-1-58023-429-0 **$8.99**

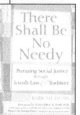

Conscience
The Duty to Obey and the Duty to Disobey
By Rabbi Harold M. Schulweis
Examines the idea of conscience and the role conscience plays in our relationships
to government, law, ethics, religion, human nature, God—and to each other.
6 x 9, 160 pp, Quality PB, 978-1-58023-419-1 **$16.99**; HC, 978-1-58023-375-0 **$19.99**

Judaism and Justice
The Jewish Passion to Repair the World
By Rabbi Sidney Schwarz; Foreword by Ruth Messinger
Explores the relationship between Judaism, social justice and the Jewish identity
of American Jews. 6 x 9, 352 pp, Quality PB, 978-1-58023-353-8 **$19.99**

Spirituality / Women's Interest

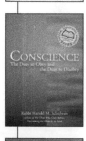

New Jewish Feminism
Probing the Past, Forging the Future
Edited by Rabbi Elyse Goldstein; Foreword by Anita Diamant
Looks at the growth and accomplishments of Jewish feminism and what they
mean for Jewish women today and tomorrow.
6 x 9, 480 pp, HC, 978-1-58023-359-0 **$24.99**

The Divine Feminine in Biblical Wisdom Literature
Selections Annotated & Explained
Translation & Annotation by Rabbi Rami Shapiro
5½ x 8½, 240 pp, Quality PB, 978-1-59473-109-9 **$16.99**
(A book from SkyLight Paths, Jewish Lights' sister imprint)

The Quotable Jewish Woman
Wisdom, Inspiration & Humor from the Mind & Heart
Edited by Elaine Bernstein Partnow
6 x 9, 496 pp, Quality PB, 978-1-58023-236-4 **$19.99**

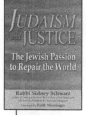

The Women's Haftarah Commentary
New Insights from Women Rabbis on the 54 Weekly Haftarah Portions,
the 5 Megillot & Special Shabbatot
Edited by Rabbi Elyse Goldstein
Illuminates the historical significance of female portrayals in the Haftarah and the
Five Megillot. 6 x 9, 560 pp, Quality PB, 978-1-58023-371-2 **$19.99**

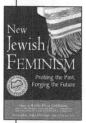

The Women's Torah Commentary
New Insights from Women Rabbis on the 54 Weekly Torah Portions
Edited by Rabbi Elyse Goldstein
Over fifty women rabbis offer inspiring insights on the Torah, in a week-by-week format.
6 x 9, 496 pp, Quality PB, 978-1-58023-370-5 **$19.99**; HC, 978-1-58023-076-6 **$34.95**

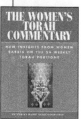

Meditation

The Magic of Hebrew Chant: Healing the Spirit, Transforming the Mind, Deepening Love
By Rabbi Shefa Gold; Foreword by Sylvia Boorstein
Introduces this transformative spiritual practice as a way to unlock the power of sacred texts and make prayer and meditation the delight of your life. Includes musical notations. 6 x 9, 352 pp, Quality PB, 978-1-58023-671-3 **$24.99**

The Magic of Hebrew Chant Companion—The Big Book of Musical Notations and Incantations
8½ x 11, 154 pp, PB, 978-1-58023-722-2 **$19.99**

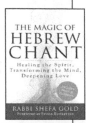

Jewish Meditation Practices for Everyday Life
Awakening Your Heart, Connecting with God
By Rabbi Jeff Roth
Offers a fresh take on meditation that draws on life experience and living life with greater clarity as opposed to the traditional method of rigorous study.
6 x 9, 224 pp, Quality PB, 978-1-58023-397-2 **$18.99**

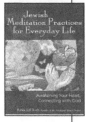

Discovering Jewish Meditation, 2nd Edition
Instruction & Guidance for Learning an Ancient Spiritual Practice
By Nan Fink Gefen, PhD 6 x 9, 208 pp, Quality PB, 978-1-58023-462-7 **$16.99**

The Handbook of Jewish Meditation Practices
A Guide for Enriching the Sabbath and Other Days of Your Life
By Rabbi David A. Cooper 6 x 9, 208 pp, Quality PB, 978-1-58023-102-2 **$16.95**

Meditation from the Heart of Judaism
Today's Teachers Share Their Practices, Techniques, and Faith
Edited by Avram Davis 6 x 9, 256 pp, Quality PB, 978-1-58023-049-0 **$16.95**

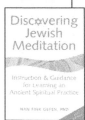

Ritual / Sacred Practices

God in Your Body: Kabbalah, Mindfulness and Embodied Spiritual Practice
By Jay Michaelson
The first comprehensive treatment of the body in Jewish spiritual practice and an essential guide to the sacred. 6 x 9, 272 pp, Quality PB, 978-1-58023-304-0 **$18.99**

The Book of Jewish Sacred Practices: CLAL's Guide to Everyday & Holiday Rituals & Blessings *Edited by Rabbi Irwin Kula and Vanessa L. Ochs, PhD*
6 x 9, 368 pp, Quality PB, 978-1-58023-152-7 **$18.95**

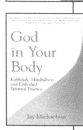

The Jewish Dream Book: The Key to Opening the Inner Meaning of Your Dreams
By Vanessa L. Ochs, PhD, with Elizabeth Ochs; Illus. by Kristina Swarner
8 x 8, 128 pp, Full-color illus., Deluxe PB w/ flaps, 978-1-58023-132-9 **$16.95**

Jewish Ritual: A Brief Introduction for Christians
By Rabbi Kerry M. Olitzky and Rabbi Daniel Judson
5½ x 8½, 144 pp, Quality PB, 978-1-58023-210-4 **$14.99**

The Rituals & Practices of a Jewish Life: A Handbook for Personal Spiritual Renewal *Edited by Rabbi Kerry M. Olitzky and Rabbi Daniel Judson*
6 x 9, 272 pp, Illus., Quality PB, 978-1-58023-169-5 **$18.95**

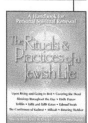

The Sacred Art of Lovingkindness: Preparing to Practice
By Rabbi Rami Shapiro 5½ x 8½, 176 pp, Quality PB, 978-1-59473-151-8 **$16.99**
(A book from SkyLight Paths, Jewish Lights' sister imprint)

Mystery & Detective Fiction

Criminal Kabbalah: An Intriguing Anthology of Jewish Mystery & Detective Fiction *Edited by Lawrence W. Raphael; Foreword by Laurie R. King*
All-new stories from twelve of today's masters of mystery and detective fiction—sure to delight mystery buffs of all faith traditions.
6 x 9, 256 pp, Quality PB, 978-1-58023-109-1 **$16.95**

Mystery Midrash: An Anthology of Jewish Mystery & Detective Fiction
Edited by Lawrence W. Raphael; Preface by Joel Siegel
6 x 9, 304 pp, Quality PB, 978-1-58023-055-1 **$16.95**

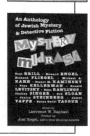

About Jewish Lights

People of all faiths and backgrounds yearn for books that attract, engage, educate, and spiritually inspire.

Our principal goal is to stimulate thought and help all people learn about who the Jewish People are, where they come from, and what the future can be made to hold. While people of our diverse Jewish heritage are the primary audience, our books speak to people in the Christian world as well and will broaden their understanding of Judaism and the roots of their own faith.

We bring to you authors who are at the forefront of spiritual thought and experience. While each has something different to say, they all say it in a voice that you can hear.

Our books are designed to welcome you and then to engage, stimulate, and inspire. We judge our success not only by whether or not our books are beautiful and commercially successful, but by whether or not they make a difference in your life.

For your information and convenience, at the back of this book we have provided a list of other Jewish Lights books you might find interesting and useful. They cover all the categories of your life:

Bar/Bat Mitzvah
Bible Study / Midrash
Children's Books
Congregation Resources
Current Events / History
Ecology / Environment
Fiction: Mystery, Science Fiction
Grief / Healing
Holidays / Holy Days
Inspiration
Kabbalah / Mysticism / Enneagram

Life Cycle
Meditation
Men's Interest
Parenting
Prayer / Ritual / Sacred Practice
Social Justice
Spirituality
Theology / Philosophy
Travel
Twelve Steps
Women's Interest

Stuart M. Matlins, Publisher